Pocket Picture Guides

AIDS

An **Essential Slide Collection of AIDS,**
based on the material in this book, is available. The
collection consists of numbered 35 mm colour
transparencies of each illustration in the book, and each
section is accompanied by a slide index for easy reference.
The material is presented in an attractive binder, which also
contains a copy of the Pocket Picture Guide. The Essential
Slide Collection is available from:

Gower Medical Publishing

Middlesex House,
34-42 Cleveland Street,
London W1P 5FB, UK.

101 5th Avenue,
New York, NY. 10003,
USA.

Pocket Picture Guides

AIDS

Ian Williams BSC,MB,MRCP(UK)

Honorary Lecturer in Genitourinary Medicine

Adrian Mindel MSC,MRCP

Senior Lecturer in Genitourinary Medicine

Ian V D Weller BSC, MD,MRCP

Reader in Genitourinary Medicine
University College and Middlesex School of Medicine
London, UK.

J.B. Lippincott Company • Philadelphia
Gower Medical Publishing • London • New York

Distributed in USA and Canada by:

J.B. Lippincott Company
East Washington Square
Philadelphia, PA 19105
USA

Distributed in UK and Continental Europe by:

Harper & Row Ltd
Middlesex House
34-42 Cleveland Street
London W1P 5FB
UK

Distributed in Japan by:

Igaku Shoin Ltd
Tokyo International
P.O. Box 5063
Tokyo
Japan

Distributed in Southeast Asia, Hong Kong,
India and Pakistan by:

Harper & Row Publishers (Asia) Pte Ltd
37 Jalal Pemimpin 02-01
Singapore 2057

Distributed in Philippines/Guam, Middle East,
Latin America and Africa by:

Harper & Row International
East Washington Square
Philadelphia, PA 19105
USA

Distributed in Australia and New Zealand by:

Harper & Row (Australasia) Pty Ltd
P.O. Box 226
Artarmon, N.S.W. 2064
Australia

Library of Congress Catalog Number: 87-82128
British Library Cataloguing in Publication Data:

Weller, Ian
    Pocket picture guides to AIDS.
    1. Man. AIDS
    1. Title II. Mindel, Adrian III,
    Williams, Ian 616.9'792

ISBN: 0-397-44578-4 (Gower/Lippincott)

PROJECT TEAM
Project Editor: Michele Campbell
Design & Illustration: Ann-Josie Down
Linework: Marion Tasker
            Mark N. Willey
Index: Gillian Lancaster
Production: Rosemary Allen
Publisher: Fiona Foley

Typeset in Sabon and Frutiger by Dawkins Typesetters Ltd.
Originated in Hong Kong by Bright Arts (HK) Ltd.
Printed in Hong Kong

PREFACE

Since the first description of the acquired immune deficiency syndrome (AIDS) in 1981 almost unprecedented progress, as far as an infectious disease is concerned, has been made. To a large extent this was because our biotechnology, in the form of molecular biology and immunological techniques, was, in a way, ready to receive the virus.

Human immunodeficiency virus (HIV) was first identified in 1983 and with the development of a permissive cell line to culture it, established as a cause in 1984. In the same year the receptor for the virus (CD4) was identified and an antibody test developed; this enabled physicians to make a serological diagnosis of infection and facilitated the screening of blood donors to reduce the risk of infection via blood products. In 1986 the first clinical trials with the antiviral agent azido-thymidine (later to become zidovudine) were begun and a variant of human immunodeficiency virus, now known as HIV-2, was isolated.

In 1987 recombinant proteins, which are now being used as candidate vaccines, were developed and in the same year it was shown that zidovudine significantly decreased mortality and the incidence of opportunistic infections, improved symptoms and CD4$^+$ lymphocyte counts, and produced an antiviral effect as measured by decrease in serum P24 protein in patients with symptomatic disease. This year zidovudine trials have begun in asymptomatic patients and recombinant CD4 is being assessed as an antiviral agent.

In spite of this progress, however, the management of persons infected with HIV tests the basic skills of the physician, particularly with respect to sensitive history taking and thorough clinical examination. These together with advances in diagnostic laboratory techniques should facilitate the early diagnosis and management of the opportunistic conditions which may cause profound disability or even threaten life. We and our patients hope that this simple atlas will in some way assist clinicians in the day-to-day care of those infected with HIV.

IVDW
AM
IW
London

CONTENTS

Preface V

Epidemiology, pathogenesis and virology
  of HIV 1

Acute and chronic manifestations
  of HIV infection 23

Kaposi's sarcoma and other tumours 43

The opportunistic infections 60

Antiviral agents and vaccines 96

Index 108

EPIDEMIOLOGY, PATHOGENESIS AND VIROLOGY OF HIV

Epidemiology

In 1981, following reports from a number of clinicians, the Centers for Disease Control (CDC) in the USA identified an outbreak of an unusual syndrome in homosexual men. This consisted of *Pneumocystis carinii* pneumonia and an aggressive form of Kaposi's sarcoma associated with an acquired immunodeficiency; it became known as acquired immunodeficiency syndrome (AIDS). Since then, the spectrum of the syndrome has widened to include other tumours, such as lymphomas, and a wide variety of opportunistic viral, bacterial, fungal and protozoal infections. Without a specific marker for the disease, an all-encompassing definition was required for case notification. The definition was modified in June 1985 with the development of routine assays for antibodies to the causative agent (Fig. 1), now termed human immunodeficiency virus (HIV), to include other tumours and conditions. It was further modified in 1987, for surveillance of AIDS cases, to include other serious manifestations of HIV disease and to take into account changes in clinical practice, such as the presumptive diagnosis of certain conditions.

EVIDENCE FOR HIV AS THE CAUSE OF AIDS AND RELATED SYNDROMES

Seroepidemiology

Prospective studies: infection antedates disease expression

Virus isolation in AIDS and related conditions

Biological plausibility: retrovirus with CD4 tropism

Human → human transmission and later disease development

? Immunization prevents infection and disease

Fig. 1 Evidence for HIV as the cause of AIDS and related syndromes.

AIDS definition (with 1987 revision)
A case of AIDS is defined as an illness characterized by one or more of the indicator diseases, depending on the status of laboratory evidence of HIV infection (Figs 2 & 3).

INDICATOR DISEASES WITHOUT LAB. EVIDENCE OF HIV

Candidiasis — oesophageal, pulmonary

Cryptococcosis — extrapulmonary

Cytomegalovirus disease — disseminated

Cryptosporidiosis – diarrhoea persisting >1 month

Herpes simplex virus (HSV) infection
— mucocutaneous ulceration lasting > 1 month
— pulmonary, oesophageal involvement

Kaposi's sarcoma — patient < 60 years of age

Primary cerebral lymphoma — patient < 60 years of age

Lymphoid interstitial pneumonia — child < 13 years of age

Mycobacterium avium
Mycobacterium kansasii } disseminated

Pneumocystis carinii pneumonia

Progressive multifocal leukoencephalopathy

Cerebral toxoplasmosis

Fig. 2 AIDS indicator diseases. In the absence of another cause of immunodeficiency and without laboratory evidence of HIV infection (patient not tested or inconclusive results), the diseases listed, when diagnosed definitively, are diagnostic of AIDS.

INDICATOR DISEASES IN PRESENCE OF LAB. EVIDENCE OF HIV

diseases diagnosed definitively

Recurrent/multiple bacterial infections — child < 13 years of age

Coccidioidomycosis — disseminated

HIV encephalopathy

Histoplasmosis — disseminated

Isosporiasis — diarrhoea persisting > 1 month

Kaposi's sarcoma at any age

Primary cerebral lymphoma at any age

Non-Hodgkin's lymphoma — diffuse, undifferentiated B cell type, or unknown phenotype

Any disseminated mycobacterial disease other than *M. tuberculosis*

Mycobacterial tuberculosis — extrapulmonary

Salmonella septicaemia — recurrent

HIV wasting syndrome

diseases diagnosed presumptively

Candidiasis — oesophageal

Cytomegalovirus retinitis with visual loss

Kaposi's sarcoma

Lymphoid interstitial pneumonia — child < 13 years of age

Mycobacterial disease (acid-fast bacilli; species not identified by culture) — disseminated

Pneumocystis carinii pneumonia

Cerebral toxoplasmosis

Fig. 3 AIDS indicator diseases. Regardless of the presence of other causes of immunodeficiency and with laboratory evidence of HIV infection, the above diseases, in addition to those listed in Fig. 2, are diagnostic of AIDS.

In the USA homosexual men still comprise about 66 percent of the total number of cases. Other groups at risk soon became apparent (Fig. 4), namely: heterosexual intravenous drug abusers; haemophiliacs and other recipients of blood

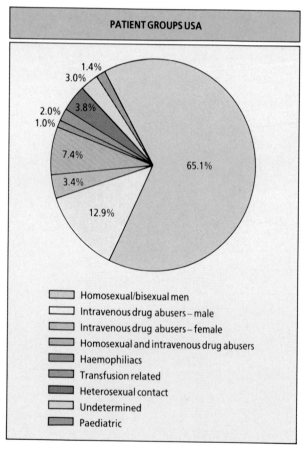

PATIENT GROUPS USA

1.4%
3.0%
3.8%
2.0%
1.0%
7.4%
3.4%
12.9%
65.1%

☐ Homosexual/bisexual men
☐ Intravenous drug abusers – male
☐ Intravenous drug abusers – female
☐ Homosexual and intravenous drug abusers
☐ Haemophiliacs
☐ Transfusion related
☐ Heterosexual contact
☐ Undetermined
☐ Paediatric

Fig. 4 Patient groups in the USA. 7% of adult cases are female and 93% male; a ratio of 1:13.5. In the heterosexual contact group the ratio is 1:1. Amongst heterosexuals who were born in the USA, 66% of cases were partners of intravenous drug abusers and 14% of bisexuals. The undetermined group are cases in whom information is incomplete, for example because of death or refusal to be interviewed.

or blood products; the heterosexual sexual partners of in-travenous drug abusers; bisexual men; prostitutes; and infants born to mothers with AIDS or in AIDS risk groups (Fig. 5).

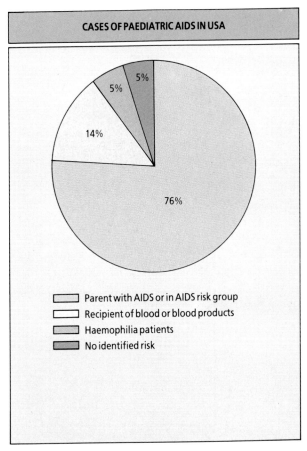

CASES OF PAEDIATRIC AIDS IN USA

5%
5%
14%
76%

☐ Parent with AIDS or in AIDS risk group
☐ Recipient of blood or blood products
☐ Haemophilia patients
☐ No identified risk

Fig. 5 Cases of paediatric AIDS in the USA.

In Europe, a further risk group was identified following reports of AIDS in Belgian and French patients who originated from Central Africa. This reflected the appearance of the syndrome there, which has currently reached epidemic proportions, with heterosexual promiscuity being a major risk factor. All the epidemiological evidence pointed to a causative agent that was sexually, parenterally and perinatally transmitted. The number of new cases reported each year continues to increase (Fig. 6) but not now exponentially, as shown by the lengthening case doubling times.

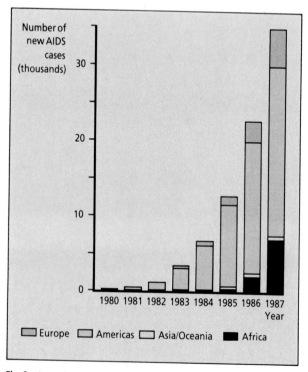

Fig. 6 Annual new cases of AIDS by world region. Modified from WHO, March 1988.

Spectrum of immune dysfunction

In AIDS patients a depletion and/or impaired function of the T helper lymphocyte stood out as a possible primary abnormality. These cells have a surface glycoprotein called CD4 (CD = cluster differentiation). A virus which was tropic for $CD4^+$ lymphocytes and which produced a cytopathic effect *in vivo* and/or disturbance of $CD4^+$ function would also produce, as secondary phenomena, many of the immune abnormalities (Fig. 7) that were described in patients with AIDS and related syndromes.

SPECTRUM OF IMMUNE DYSFUNCTION

Lymphopenia: ↓ T helper ($CD4^+$)

Skin anergy

↓ Proliferative responses (mitogens, antigens, alloantigens)

Cytotoxic responses
    ↓ cytotoxic T cell ($CD8^+$)
    ↓ natural killer cell

↓ Monocyte function

↑ Immunoglobulins
    ↑ polyclonal B cell activation
    ↓ primary antibody response

↑ Circulating immune complexes
    ↑ Autoantibodies
    ↑ acid-labile interferon
    ↑ β_2 microglobulin
    ↑ alpha-1-thymosin

Fig. 7 Spectrum of immune dysfunction.

The CD4$^+$ lymphocyte is an ideal target for an infectious agent intent on compromising a host's immune response. It has a pivotal role in the development of an adequate response to a foreign antigen, particularly an intracellular one (Fig. 8). CD4$^+$ lymphocytes are triggered by antigen presented by macrophages (antigen-presenting cells) in association with class II antigens of the major histocompatibility complex (MHC). Contact with the macrophage, and the influence of soluble proteins released by it, for example interleukin-1 and interferon γ, results in activation of the CD4$^+$ subset. The latter stimulate the differentiation and maturation of other T cells, namely the CD8$^+$ subset, which includes specific cytotoxic T cells (which eliminate cells displaying antigen in association with class I MHC proteins on the membrane of the infected target cell), and suppressor T cells, which later dampen down the immune response. The CD4$^+$ lymphocyte helps in the proliferation and differentiation of antigen-specific B cells, with subsequent production of antibody. The production of antibody enables killer cells, which are responsible for antibody-dependent cell cytotoxicity (ADCC), to destroy the infected target cell. CD4$^+$ cells also activate natural killer cells and macrophages. The effects of CD4$^+$ lymphocytes are mediated by direct contact and by the influence of lymphokines such as interferon γ and interleukin-2.

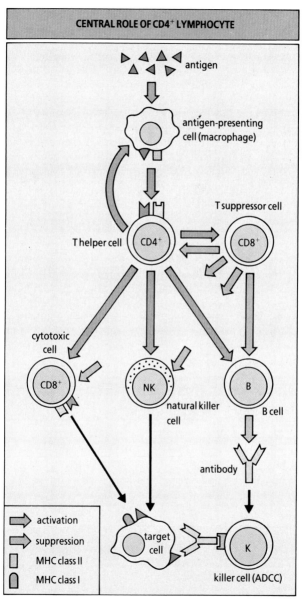

CENTRAL ROLE OF CD4⁺ LYMPHOCYTE

Fig. 8 The central role of the CD4⁺ lymphocyte in the development of reponse to antigen.

The virus

Animal retroviruses are known to cause a variety of tumours, immunodeficiency and autoimmune diseases. Infection with a human T lymphotropic retrovirus, originally termed human T cell leukaemia virus (HTLV) but now called human T lymphotropic virus type I (HTLV-I), was known to be associated with an adult T cell leukaemia and was endemic in Japan, the Caribbean, and parts of the USA, Africa and Italy. A second, closely related virus, HTLV-II, has been isolated from a single patient with leukaemia but has not yet been conclusively associated with any human disease. Both retroviruses are tropic for $CD4^+$ cells and transform them *in vitro*.

In 1983, a group of French investigators working on a lymphocyte culture from a patient with PGL identified a retrovirus which they called lymphadenopathy associated virus (LAV). Similar viruses were identified in patients with AIDS. In 1984, two American groups also independently identified similar viruses, which were termed HTLV-III by investigators at the National Institutes of Health (NIH) (who had also discovered HTLV-I and -II) and AIDS-related retrovirus (ARV) by the group in San Francisco. These all represented isolates of the same virus, namely HIV (Figs 9 & 10).

Demonstration of HIV

The virus may be demonstrated by:
- electronmicroscopy
- cytopathic effect in permissive cells
- expressed antigens on permissive cells using immuno-fluorescence
- reverse transcriptase enzyme activity in supernatants
- antigen assays
- viral DNA/RNA using nucleic acid probes

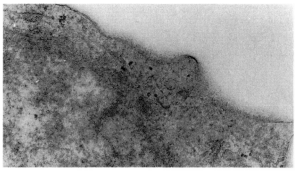

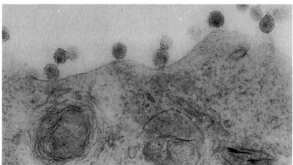

Fig. 9 HIV has a diameter of 100–120nm. The virions have a cylindrical core on electron microscopy. Complete virions are released from infected cells by characteristic budding, as shown here.

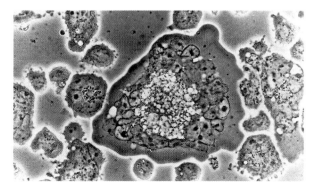

Fig. 10 The virus is tropic for CD4$^+$ cells and produces a cytopathic effect in T cell cultures with cell fusion and formation of multinucleate giant cells, as seen here, followed by cell death.

A permanent virus-producing cell line was initially difficult to obtain. However, the group at NIH achieved this with a T cell line which was permissive and partially resistant to the cytopathic effect of the virus. This made available viral anti-

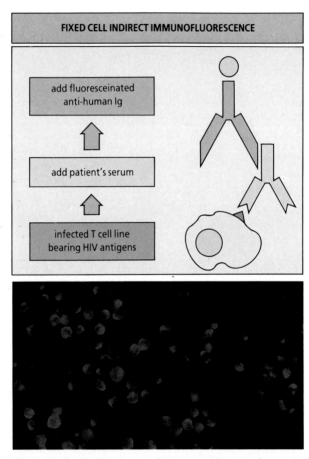

FIXED CELL INDIRECT IMMUNOFLUORESCENCE

add fluoresceinated anti-human Ig

↑

add patient's serum

↑

infected T cell line bearing HIV antigens

Fig. 11 Fixed cell indirect immunofluorescence. The patient's serum is incubated with an HIV-infected T cell line (CEM,CBL); any HIV antibodies present in the serum will bind to HIV antigens on the T cells (upper). Unbound proteins are washed away. Bound HIV antibodies are detected by adding anti-human immunoglobulin tagged with fluoresceinated isothiocyanate (FITC), which fluoresces green under ultraviolet light (lower).

gens, which allowed for the development of assays for specific antibodies (Figs 11–15), which proved invaluable in early and later epidemiological surveys.

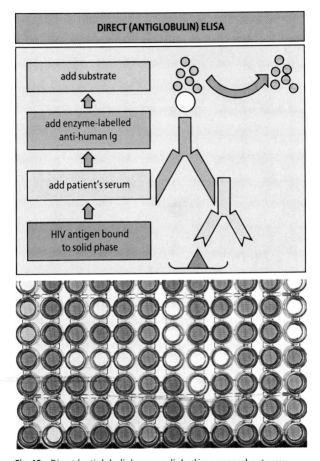

Fig. 12 Direct (antiglobulin) enzyme-linked immunosorbent assay (ELISA). The patient's serum is added to antigen, which is bound to a microtitre plate well (upper). Any HIV antibodies present in the serum will bind to antigen. These antibodies are detected using an anti-human Ig coupled to an enzyme (in this case, horseradish peroxidase), which converts an added substrate to a coloured end product (yellow in this example). A developed plate is shown (lower). The amount of anti-HIV present is measured by optical density scanning of the well.

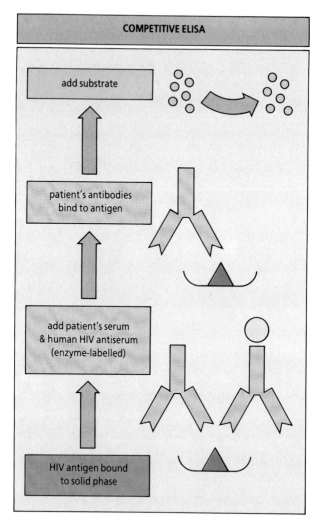

Fig. 13 Competitive ELISA. The patient's serum is added to HIV antigen bound to a microtitre plate well. Any anti-HIV antibodies present will compete with the added HIV antiserum, which has been coupled with an enzyme (horseradish peroxidase), for antigen binding. Anti-HIV in the patient's serum will be preferentially bound to the antigen, resulting in no conversion of the substrate to its coloured end product.

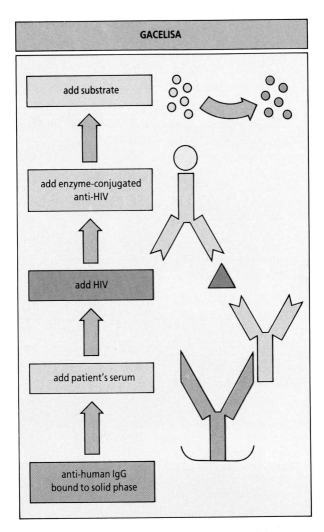

GACELISA

add substrate

add enzyme-conjugated anti-HIV

add HIV

add patient's serum

anti-human IgG bound to solid phase

Fig. 14 IgG capture ELISA (GACELISA). A diluted sample of the patient's serum is incubated with anti-human globulin (class-specific IgG) absorbed onto a solid phase, such as a microtitre well. After washing, HIV antigen is added; this will bind to any antibodies captured by the anti-human globulin. Binding of antigen is detected by addition of an enzyme-conjugated anti-virus antibody. These assays are more sensitive when used on body fluids e.g. saliva, in which antibody concentrations are lower than in serum.

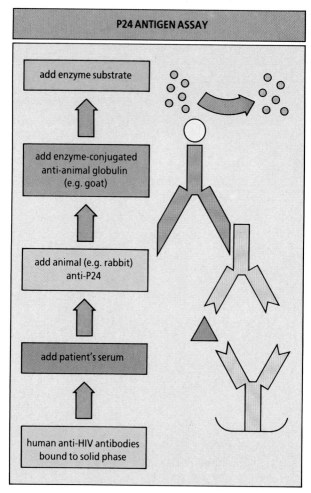

Fig. 15 Antigen assay. An ELISA has been developed to detect the presence of the viral protein, P24, in serum. The patient's serum is added to a solid phase (e.g. polystyrene beads) coated with human anti-HIV antibody; this will bind any HIV antigen present in the serum to the solid phase. Following washing of unbound proteins anti-P24 is added, which binds to any HIV-24 antigen present. Bound anti-P24 is detected by adding an anti-animal globulin conjugated with horseradish peroxidase, which converts an added substrate to a coloured end product. P24 is a laboratory prognostic marker and is useful for monitoring antiviral therapy.

A high prevalence of anti-HIV was demonstrated in patients with AIDS and at risk of AIDS compared to controls. The increasing prevalence of anti-HIV and AIDS in the UK and other countries in Europe followed, after a period of three to four years, the pattern already evident in the USA (Figs 16 & 17). In prospective studies the presence of anti-HIV was shown to antedate both the development of AIDS and its related syndromes. HIV can be demonstrated in lymphocyte cultures from the majority of patients with anti-HIV. Sera from anti-HIV positive individuals at various stages of infection have only weak neutralizing activity *in vitro*.

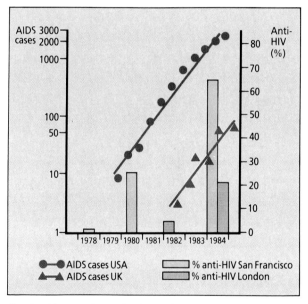

Fig. 16 Rising prevalence of anti-HIV in homosexual men attending STD clinics in the USA and UK. AIDS cases are recorded by 6 month period of report.

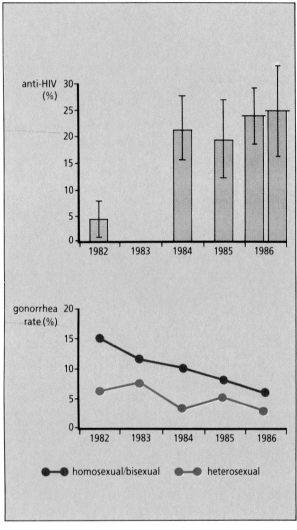

Fig. 17 A slower rise in the prevalence of anti-HIV since 1984 has been documented amongst homosexual and bisexual men attending a London STD clinic (upper). This, together with a fall in the annual rate of gonorrhoea among London men (lower), indicates a significant swing towards safer sexual practices.

CD4$^+$ Tropism

Only cells bearing or producing the CD4$^+$ antigen are susceptible to infection by HIV (Fig. 18). The expression of the antigen is not restricted to T helper cells but is also displayed on monocytes and macrophages and some B cell lines. *In vivo* infection of macrophages further amplifies its effects on the immune system. Cells in the brains of AIDS patients have also been demonstrated to contain HIV genomes. Microglial cells are good candidates for infection.

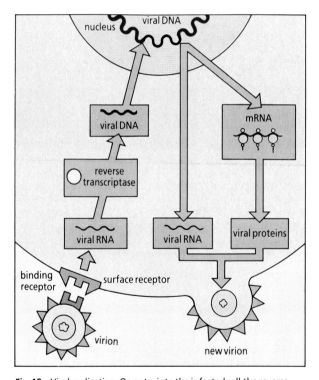

Fig. 18 Viral replication. On entry into the infected cell, the reverse transcriptase enzyme makes a DNA copy (proviral DNA) of the RNA genome. Infected cells can contain both unintegrated and integrated proviral DNA. The latter allows for latent non-productive viral infection. During productive replication, RNA transcripts are made from proviral DNA and complete virions are assembled and released from the infected cells.

Genetic Structure

Molecular cloning and analysis of the nucleotide sequence of the genome reveals that HIV is distinct from HTLV-I and-II. It has the basic structures common to all retroviruses, namely three genes – the *gag, pol* and *env* genes (Fig.19) – which code for the core, reverse transcriptase (polymerase) and envelope proteins respectively. These are flanked by long terminal repeat (LTR) sequences, which have an important regulatory role in viral gene expression. In addition to these genes there are areas containing open reading frames (ORFs); these contain a number of genes which encode proteins, which in turn intricately control the expression of viral genes. Comparison of different isolates of HIV have shown that there is genomic diversity. This seems to be most marked in the *env* gene region coding for the envelope glycoprotein, in which potential antigens involved in virus neutralization may reside. More recently, viruses have been isolated from both patients and healthy subjects in West Africa: these are genetically more similar to simian T cell lymphotropic virus (STLV-III), now known as simian immunodeficiency virus (SIV), than are the previous human retrovirus isolates (HIV-1). SIV is present in African green monkeys across equatorial Africa and causes an AIDS-like disease in captive rhesus monkeys; further work on this and other primate viruses will provide important clues to the origin of HIV. The human isolates were termed HTLV-IV and LAV-2 according to the allegiances of the groups who discovered them, but are now known as HIV-2.

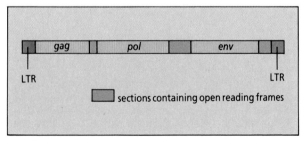

Fig. 19 Genetic structure of HIV.

HIV Proteins

If HIV virions are disrupted and examined by polyacrylamide gel electrophoresis, a number of different proteins are revealed. Proteins separated in this way can be used to detect antibodies in patients' sera to individual viral proteins (the basis of the western blot technique) (Fig.20). The envelope proteins are heavily glycosylated and are of high molecular weight. A glycoprotein (GP) of 160,000 (160k) molecular weight is the precursor of the major envelope glycoprotein, GP120k (Fig.21) and a smaller hydrophobic nonglycosylated protein, GP41k, which represents the portion of the envelope protein which is inserted into the inner membrane of the virus (transmembrane protein).

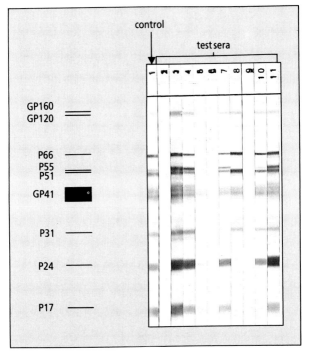

Fig. 20 Antibodies to viral proteins in patients' sera demonstrated using the western blot technique. Line 1 is a positive control.

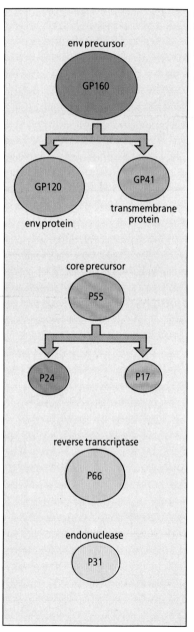

Fig. 21 Viral proteins. Recent work suggests that GP120 is the viral envelope component which interacts with the CD4$^+$ receptor.

ACUTE AND CHRONIC MANIFESTATIONS OF HIV INFECTION

The spectrum of disease produced by HIV infection is wide. A simple classification system devised by the Centre for Disease Control in Atlanta, USA illustrates the different stages of infection and the variety of clinical problems seen (Fig. 22). The pathogenesis of disease is multifactorial, ranging from syndromes caused directly by HIV infection to those which reflect the deleterious effect of HIV on the patient's immune system. Major opportunistic infections and tumours in severely immunocompromized patients are discussed in later sections.

CDC CLASSIFICATION
I : Acute Infection
II : Asymptomatic
III : Persistent Generalized Lymphadenopathy

IV : Other Disease
A   Constitutional disease
B   Neurological disease: dementia, myelopathy, peripheral neuropathy
C   Secondary infectious diseases
  C1 Specified in CDC surveillance definition of AIDS
  C2 Other infections: – oral hairy leukoplakia
             – multidermatomal herpes zoster
             – nocardiosis
             – oral candidiasis
             – tuberculosis
D   Secondary cancers: specified in CDC surveillance definition of AIDS
E   Other conditions: e.g. chronic lymphocytic interstitial pneumonitis, patients with constitutional disease not fulfilling IV A, other infections or tumours not listed in IV C1 or IV D.

Fig. 22   CDC classification of spectrum of disease produced by HIV infection.

ACUTE SEROCONVERSION ILLNESSES
Glandular Fever-Like-Illness
fevers
rash
arthralgia
lymphadenopathy
Neurological Syndromes
aseptic meningitis
acute encephalitis
myelopathy
neuropathy

Fig. 23 Acute seroconversion illnesses. Investigations should be structured to exclude other possible causes before acute infection with HIV is considered. The symptoms reflect an acute viraemia with HIV. The CD4$^+$ to CD8$^+$ ratio is reduced due to a rise in circulating CD8$^+$ cells.

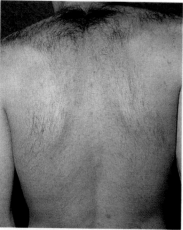

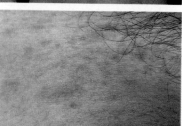

Fig. 24 Exanthema of acute infection. A diffuse macular rash on the trunk, which was also present on the face. This patient was HIV antibody-negative but core antigen (P24)-positive at presentation, one month later he became HIV antibody-positive. A thrombocytopenia was noted at the time of the acute illness.

Acute Infection

A non-specific viral or glandular-fever-like illness occurs at seroconversion in a minority of patients (Figs 23 & 24). Rarely, acute neurological syndromes are seen; these include encephalitis, aseptic meningitis, myelopathy and neuropathy.

An incubation period of 1–6 weeks occurs before onset of symptoms. HIV antibodies are generally detected 4–12 weeks after initial exposure (Fig. 25). Diagnosis is confirmed by testing an acute phase and convalescent serum for HIV antibodies. In view of the implications — medical, social and psychological — of a positive diagnosis, the possibility should be fully discussed with the patient and consent sought to carry out HIV serological tests. An acute viraemia may be detected before the appearance of antibodies by assaying for an HIV core protein (P24).

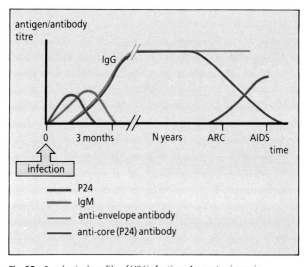

Fig. 25 Serological profile of HIV infection. An acute viraemia, detected by the presence of P24 core antigen precedes the appearance of weak neutralizing antibodies (IgG and IgM) to the 'whole' virus. Whilst the patient remains asymptomatic high titres of antibodies to envelope and core proteins persist and core antigen remains detectable in only a minority of patients. As immunodeficiency develops the anti-P24 titre falls but antibodies to the envelope (GP 41, 120, 160) remain elevated. P24 core antigenaemia recurs with time and is found in 50–60% of patients with ARC and AIDS.

Chronic Infection

As far as is known, all patients exposed to a significant inoculum of virus will remain infected. The natural history of chronic infection spans many years with the development of AIDS as an endpoint. In the early phase of infection the majority of patients are well and asymptomatic, the only evidence of infection being a positive HIV antibody test; management at this stage involves dealing with mainly social and psychological problems. On examination, a degree of lymphadenopathy is found. One third of patients fulfil the definition for persistent generalized lymphadenopathy

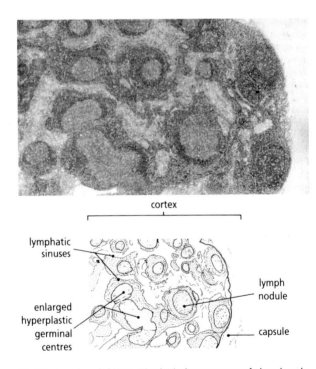

cortex

lymphatic sinuses

enlarged hyperplastic germinal centres

lymph nodule

capsule

Fig. 26 Lymph node biopsy. Histological appearances of a lymph node from a patient with PGL showing the typical finding of follicular hyperplasia. This is non-specific for HIV infection and is commonly seen in other reactive lymphadenopathies Courtesy of Dr D Katz.

(PGL) with nodes of at least 1cm in diameter at two extrainguinal sites for three months or more. The nodes are symmetrical, mobile and non-tender and show follicular hyperplasia (Fig. 26) on histological examination. Referral for lymph node biopsy is indicated only if the lymphadenopathy is markedly asymmetrical, if the nodes are tender or rapidly enlarging, if enlarged hilar nodes or hepatosplenomegaly are evident, or if constitutional symptoms such as fever and weight loss are present. In such cases the diagnoses of mycobacterial infections, lymphoma or lymph node involvement with Kaposi's sarcoma need to be excluded.

As patients become immunocompromized, many complain of constitutional symptoms. These vary from mild fatigue to debilitating diarrhoea, night sweats and fevers. These may appear as a prelude to a major opportunistic infection and form part of the syndrome known as AIDS-related complex (ARC) (Fig. 27), which is in part covered by stage IV A of the CDC classification.

The clinical sequelae of chronic infection are commonly seen on the skin, in the oropharynx, in the nervous system and in the blood. Many of these are often the first indicators of a depressed cellular immune system.

AIDS RELATED COMPLEX (ARC)

Fever persisting > 1 month
Weight loss of 10% baseline within 3 months } CDC IV A
Diarrhoea persisting > 1 month
Fatigue — reducing physical activity
Unexplained night sweats
Oral candida — CDC IV C2
Oral hairy leukoplakia — CDC IV C2
Herpes zoster within 3 months
Persistent generalized lymphadenopathy

Fig. 27 AIDS Related Complex (ARC). A combination of 2 or more of the above signs and symptoms for 3 months or longer constitutes ARC and preludes the onset of AIDS. Constitutional symptoms are attributed to HIV only in the absence of a concurrent illness or condition to explain them.

Skin

Skin problems (Fig. 28) are seen at all stages of chronic infection. Patients with PGL may complain of dry skin or of a generalized folliculitis (Figs 29 & 30).

CHRONIC MANIFESTATIONS OF HIV INFECTION IN THE SKIN/OROPHARYNX
Skin
Viral Herpes simplex (type 1 & 2) — anogenital Varicella zoster Human papilloma virus Molluscum contagiosum
Fungi Tinea cruris/pedis/corporis/other Candidiasis — interdigital, perianal Pityriasis versicolor
Bacterial Folliculitis — mild, severe, acneiform Impetigo
Other Seborrhoeic dermatitis Psoriasis
Oropharynx

Candidiasis
Hairy leukoplakia
Aphthous ulcers
Herpes simplex
Dental disease
  — periodontitis
  — abscesses
  — necrotizing ulcerative gingivitis

Fig. 28 Chronic manifestations of HIV infection in the skin and oropharynx.

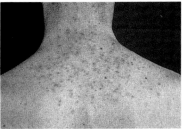

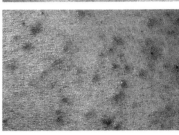

Fig. 29 Folliculitis. Diffuse folliculitis in a patient with PGL. Skin disinfectant and cleansing solutions are helpful, as is treatment with a prolonged course of low-dose antibiotics.

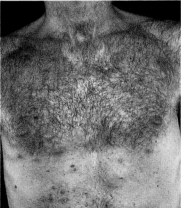

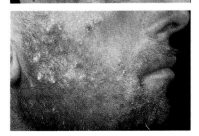

Fig. 30 Folliculitis. Upper: acneiform eruption in a patient with AIDS. Lower: severe folliculitis of the face involving mainly the beard area. Courtesy of The Institute of Dermatology.

As patients progress, seborrhoeic dermatitis (Fig 31) and many minor opportunistic infections occur, the most common of which are herpes simplex (Figs 32 & 33) dermatophyte infections (Figs 34 & 35) and varicella zoster eruptions (Fig. 36).

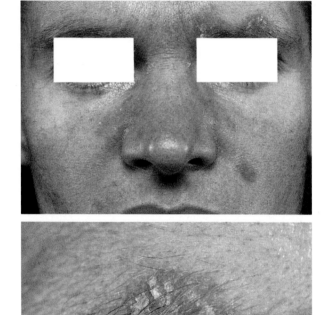

Fig. 31 Seborrhoeic dermatitis. Upper: the facial distribution has been likened to a butterfly rash but patches also occur in the eyebrows, hairline and postauricular areas. Lower: this patch is characteristically erythematous with overlying greasy scales. The condition is occasionally confused with psoriasis (see Fig. 39)

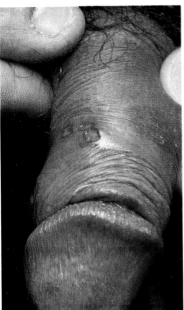

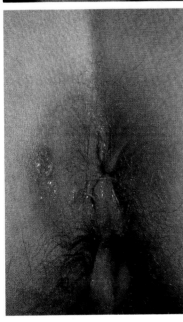

Fig. 32 Herpes simplex. Upper: genital herpes. Multiple, painful lesions often coalesce into superficial shallow ulcers. Lower: perianal herpes. Perianal HSV infection is common and often recurs. Large persistent mucocutaneous ulcers are diagnostic of AIDS. Prophylactic treatment with acyclovir is often needed.

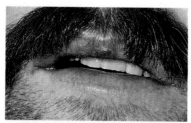

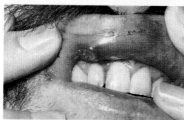

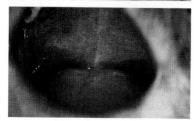

Fig. 33 Herpes simplex. Upper and middle: labial HSV infection. Lower: HSV infection of the fauces and palate.

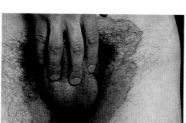

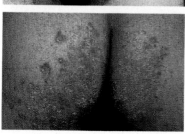

Fig. 34 Fungal infections. Tinea cruris in two different patients. Fig. 34 lower by courtesy of The Institute of Dermatology.

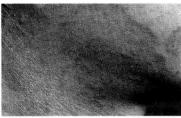

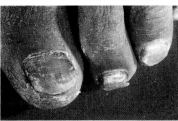

Fig. 35 Fungal infections. Upper: tinea corporis. Lower: chronic dermatophyte infection of the nail and interdigital involvement in a patient with AIDS.

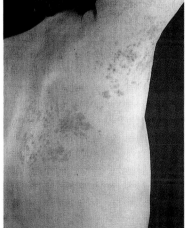

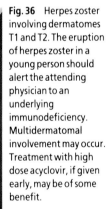

Fig. 36 Herpes zoster involving dermatomes T1 and T2. The eruption of herpes zoster in a young person should alert the attending physician to an underlying immunodeficiency. Multidermatomal involvement may occur. Treatment with high dose acyclovir, if given early, may be of some benefit.

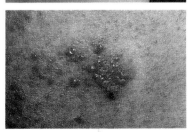

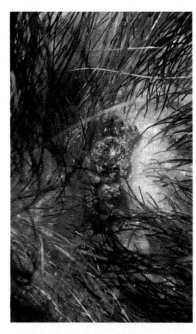

Fig. 37 Human papillomavirus (HPV) infection. Wart on the chin of a patient with PGL. Problems with mucocutaneous warts are not normally severe.

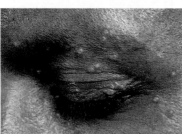

Fig. 38 Molluscum contagiosum. Lesions commonly occur on the face and neck. They appear as pearly-white umbilicated nodules. The condition is caused by infection with a pox virus; treatment is difficult.

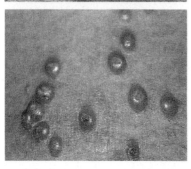

Other viral infections of the skin include human papilloma virus infection (Fig. 37) and molluscum contagiosum (Fig. 38). Several reports suggest that there is an increased incidence of psoriasis in patients with chronic HIV infection (Fig. 39).

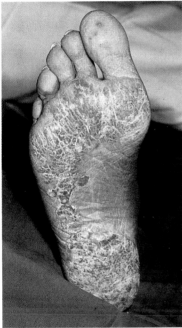

Fig. 39 Psoriasis. Upper: psoriasis on the foot of patient with AIDS. Lower: typical appearance of a patch of psoriasis.

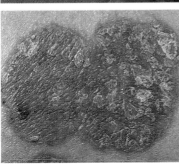

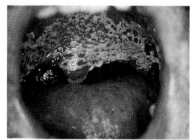

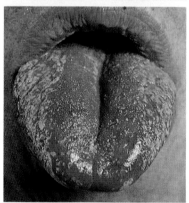

Fig. 40 Oral candidiasis. Severe oral candidiasis, as seen here, represents progression to stage IV C2 disease.

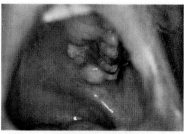

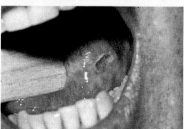

Fig. 41 Aphthous mouth ulcers. Upper: large aphthous ulcer of the alveolar ridge. Lower: chronic aphthous ulcer of the tongue. These are troublesome but may respond to steroid lozenges or paste. Other causes, such as HSV infection, should be excluded.

Oropharynx

Frequently, the first clinical presentation of a severely suppressed immune system is oral candidiasis (Fig. 40), which tends to recur following therapy. Aphthous ulcers (Fig. 41) both small and large, can occur, and may cause much discomfort. Dental problems include periodontitis and necrotizing ulcerative gingivitis (Fig. 42)

Hairy leukoplakia (Fig. 43) appears to be found only in patients with chronic HIV infection. It occurs on the lateral border of the tongue and is thought to be due to infection with Epstein-Barr virus. The lesion may come and go; and is associated with a higher incidence of progression to AIDS.

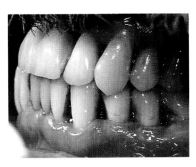

Fig. 42 HIV related gingivitis. Typical case showing gum recession and ulceration. A course of metronidazole is helpful. Courtesy of Dr D Cornick.

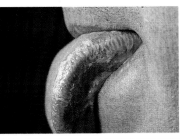

Fig. 43 Hairy leukoplakia. Typical appearances of oral hairy leukoplakia, an early sign of stage IV (C2) disease associated with a high risk of progression to AIDS. Treatment is not normally necessary.

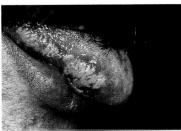

Haematology

Haematological abnormalities occur in patients with PGL, ARC and AIDS. A varying degree of anaemia and/or leukopenia is seen. Red cell morphology is not distinctive, and the anaemia is normochromic and normocytic. A combination of factors such as chronic illness, intercurrent infection, malnutrition, immune cytopenias, drugs and direct HIV infection, may be responsible.

A neutropenia and/or lymphopenia causes the overall leukopenia. The lymphopenia broadly mirrors the fall in the $CD4^+$ cell count, which occurs with time. The neutropenia is thought to be the result of an autoimmune mechanism with anti-neutrophil antibodies or immune complex deposition.

Findings on examination of the bone marrow are non-specific but include variable cellularity (Figs 44 & 45) and erythroid and myeloid dysplasia. The marrow should be cultured if a disseminated opportunistic infection (e.g. mycobacterial (Fig. 46) or fungal) is suspected.

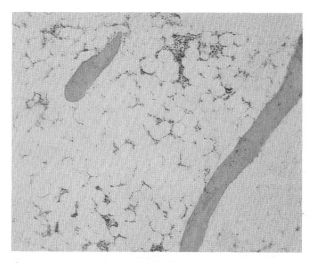

Fig. 44 Bone marrow trephine biopsy. Severe hypoplasia of all cell lines is evident. This biopsy was taken from an AIDS patient with a marked pancytopenia unrelated to drug therapy. ×100. Courtesy of Dr F Matthey and Dr H Cohen.

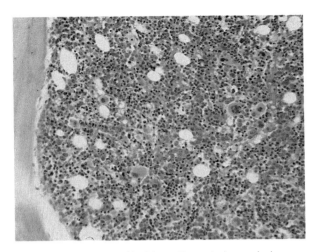

Fig. 45 Bone marrow trephine biopsy. Alternatively, a marked hypercellular marrow may be seen. This biopsy was taken from an AIDS patient who was currently taking zidovudine. A hypercellular marrow and immune cytopenias are unrelated to drug therapy. × 100. Courtesy of Dr F Matthey and Dr H Cohen.

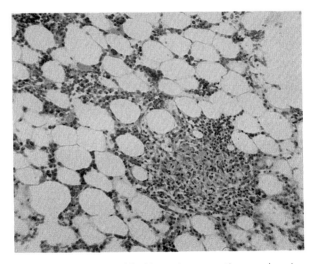

Fig. 46 Bone marrow trephine biopsy. A non-caseating granuloma is evident (right of centre field). This patient had disseminated mycobacterial tuberculosis. × 100. Courtesy of Dr F Matthey and Dr H Cohen.

An autoimmune thrombocytopenia (Fig. 47) is occasionally seen in patients with PGL and ARC. In the majority this is not severe and monitoring of the platelet count is all that is necessary; spontaneous recovery may occur. Very occasionally a severe thrombocytopenia is seen with the patient experiencing purpura (Fig. 48) and spontaneous haemorrhage. Steroids, high-dose intravenous immunoglobulin and zidovudine are used in treatment but splenectomy is often necessary in severe cases.

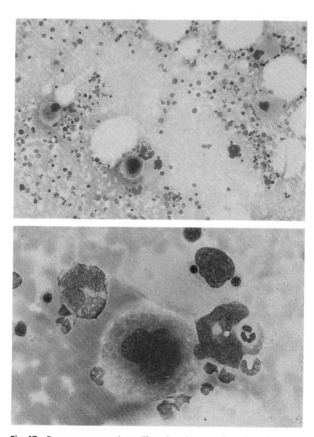

Fig. 47 Bone marrow aspirate. There is an increased number of megakaryocytes. This aspirate was taken from a patient with autoimmune thrombocytopenia. He later underwent splenectomy. ×100(upper); ×400(lower). Courtesy of Dr F Matthey and Dr H Cohen.

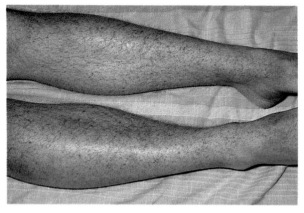

Fig. 48 Autoimmune thrombocytopenia. A generalized purpuric rash on the legs of a patient with autoimmune thrombocytopenia.

Risk of progression

Whether all HIV infected patients will progress to AIDS is not yet known. Progression rates in various cohorts of seropositive patients in the UK and North America appear to differ. Studies in San Francisco and New York, where AIDS cases were first noted, report a 3 year progression rate from asymptomatic seropositive stage to AIDS of 22% and 34% respectively, in contrast to 9% in other areas of North America.

These differences are probably explained by differences in the length of infection, the higher rates being seen in areas where HIV first appeared. Future projections suggest that about 50% of patients will have developed AIDS 10 years after seroconversion. The incidence per year in infected patients is approximately 5–7%.

Detailed longitudinal follow-up of patients has identified clinical and laboratory markers that are associated with a high risk of progression to AIDS (Fig. 49). Simple clinical and haematological markers are predictive and are commonly seen in patients with ARC. The progression rate from ARC to AIDS is about 40–50% over 2 years rising to 90% if the CD4$^+$ cell count is low.

More sophisticated serological markers are also useful and occur in patients that are otherwise asymptomatic. These abnormalities may appear years before the onset of clinical problems. Of these, an increase of β_2 microglobulin, loss of anti-P24 antibody and appearance of P24 core antigen together with a decreased PCV are the most predictive. The presence of two or more of these markers increases the risk.

The detection of prognostic markers helps to identify patients at high risk of progression. The ability to do this will be important for future evaluation and employment of early treatment.

CLINICAL AND LABORATORY MARKERS ASSOCIATED WITH AN INCREASED RISK OF PROGRESSION TO AIDS	
Clinical	
Constitutional symptoms Oral candidiasis Oral hairy leukoplakia	
Laboratory	
Simple	**Sophisticated**
Anaemia (PCV)	↓ CD4$^+$ lymphocytes
	↑ CD8$^+$ lymphocytes
Lymphopenia	↑ β_2 microglobulin
Neutropenia	↑ P24
↑ ESR	↓ anti-P24

Fig. 49 Clinical and laboratory markers associated with an increased risk of progression to AIDS.

KAPOSI'S SARCOMA AND OTHER TUMOURS

Kaposi's Sarcoma

Classical Kaposi's sarcoma (KS) is a rare tumour in North America and Europe with an annual incidence of 0.02-0.06/ 100,000. It occurs mainly in men over 50 years of age, often of Jewish or Mediterranean ancestry. It is usually confined to the lower limbs, runs an indolent course and responds well to radiotherapy or chemotherapy. The tumour also occurs in immunocompromised patients, such as renal allograft recipients, in whom it is more aggressive. Withdrawal of immunosuppression in this situation leads to tumour regression in as many as 50% of cases. Kaposi's sarcoma is also a common tumour in Central Africa where, in some areas, it accounts for 9% of all malignancies. The majority of cases are similar to the classical form previously seen in North America and Europe. A generalized variety with mucocutaneous, lymph node and visceral involvement occurs in children and young adults; this most resembles the disease seen in AIDS.

In the developed world, Kaposi's sarcoma of AIDS affects mainly young homosexual men. This group has a higher incidence of the tumour than other risk groups, who present more frequently with opportunistic infections. The median survival in AIDS patients with Kaposi's sarcoma alone is 18–24 months.

The disease in AIDS is characterized by widespread involvement of the skin (Figs 50–56), mucous membranes (Fig. 57), viscera and lymph nodes (Figs 58–59). Skin lesions are the most common presenting complaint. The gastrointestinal tract is often involved. About 50% of patients have lymph node and/or gut involvement. Involvement of the oropharynx, oesophagus, stomach (Fig. 60), duodenum and colon (Fig. 61) has been demonstrated. Lesions resemble the range seen in the skin, from small, flat telangiectatic lesions, not well demonstrated by contrast studies and only seen at endoscopy (Fig. 62), to larger nodular or polypoid lesions.

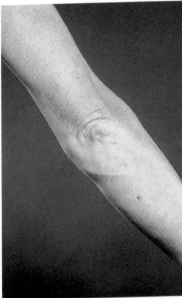

Fig.50 Early lesions of Kaposi's sarcoma. These appear as pink or red macules or papules, and may be difficult to differentiate from other skin conditions such as ecchymoses, naevi, dermatofibromata, secondary syphilis or lichen planus.

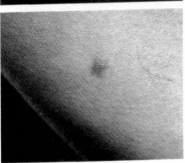

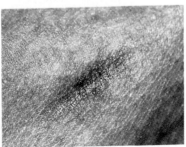

Fig.51 Later lesion of KS. The lesion is raised and may present as a violaceous plaque (as in this case) or a nodule.

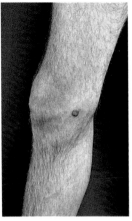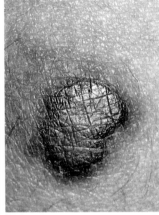

Fig.52 Later lesion of KS. Nodular presentation.

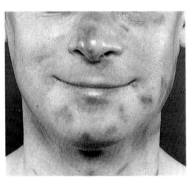

Fig.53 The later lesions are followed by disseminated skin lesions, which may appear on the face (as in this example), trunk or limbs.

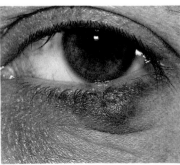

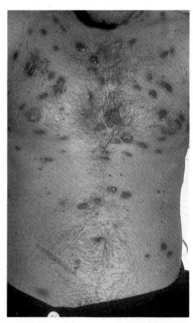

Fig.54 Disseminated skin lesions on the trunk.

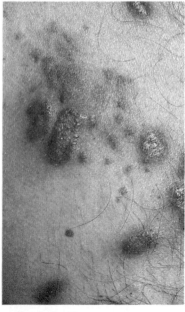

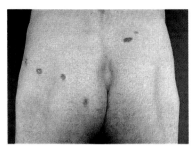

Fig.55 Disseminated skin lesions on the buttocks.

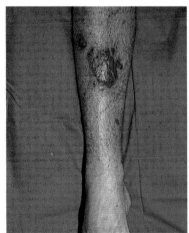

Fig.56 Disseminated skin lesions on the leg.

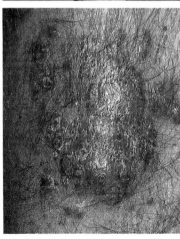

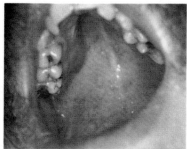

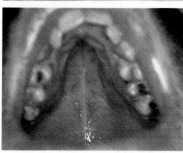

Fig.57 The mucous membranes are also involved, the palate being a common site. This case shows KS in the upper inner alveolar ridges.

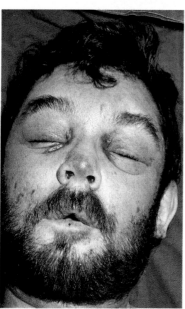

Fig.58 Marked periorbital facial oedema secondary to lymphatic involvement. Lesions are also seen on the face and nose.

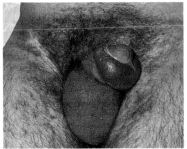

Fig.59 Oedema of the penis and scrotum as a result of pelvic and inguinal lymphatic and lymph node involvement.

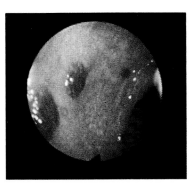

Fig.60 KS in the stomach. Three nodules seen on gastroscopy. Courtesy of Dr J Dowsett.

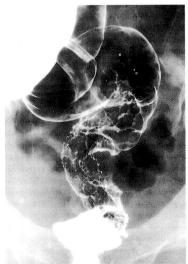

Fig.61 Barium enema: rectal Kaposi's sarcoma producing multiple filling defects.

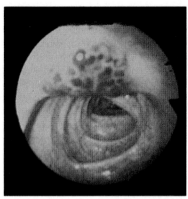

Fig.62 KS in the colon. Clusters of purple nodules seen at colonoscopy. Courtesy of Dr Alvin E Friedman-Kien.

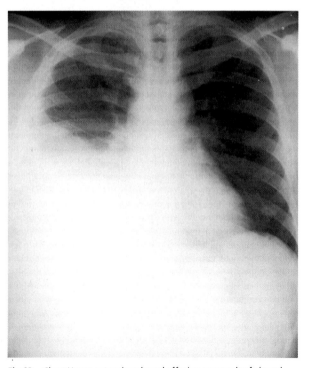

Fig.63 Chest X-ray: extensive pleural effusion as a result of pleural Kaposi's sarcoma and/or obstruction to lymphatic drainage. Treatment is difficult, as with any effusion secondary to malignancy.

Nodules of Kaposi's sarcoma also occur in the lungs. Chest X-ray appearances vary from confluent, irregular masses to interstitial nodularity (Figs. 63 & 64). CT scanning of the thorax may be useful to distinguish solid lesions (Fig. 65). On bronchoscopy, endobronchial lesions may be seen, or narrowing or obstruction of the bronchial lumen from a parenchymal Kaposi's mass may be evident.

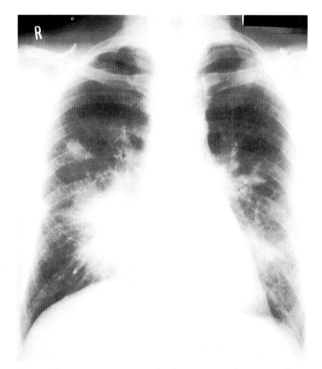

Fig.64   Chest X-ray: appearance of pulmonary Kaposi's sarcoma. There is a large right perihilar mass plus smaller nodules in the periphery. This patient also has a tracheostomy tube which was inserted as an emergency measure following acute laryngeal obstruction due to KS.

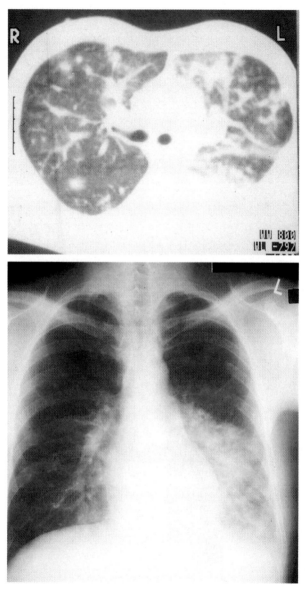

Fig.65 Upper: cross-sectional CT scan of the thorax. There are solid nodules in the lung parenchyma, especially on the left. Lower: chest X-ray appearance of the same patient. Courtesy of Professor S G Semple.

Treatment of Kaposi's sarcoma is palliative. Radiotherapy is helpful, especially around the face and neck and oropharynx (Fig. 66) where individual lesions are often disfiguring. If cutaneous lesions are widespread or if there is visceral involvement, treatment with chemotherapy or α-interferon may produce a partial remission in approximately 30–40% of patients. Histologically, established Kaposi's sarcoma consists of spindle-shaped cells arranged in nodules and broad bands, and contains vascular slits filled with extravasated erythrocytes (Figs 67a & b). The histological appearances of epidemic and classical Kaposi's sarcoma are indistinguishable. The diagnosis of Kaposi's sarcoma in very early skin lesions may be extremely difficult, based on little more than a few irregular, dilated vascular channels in the mid-dermis and a mild inflammatory cell infiltrate (Fig. 67c).

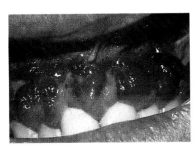
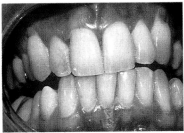

Fig.66 Upper: Kaposi's sarcoma affecting the gums. Lower: the same patient following an effective course of local radiotherapy. Courtesy of Dr D Cornick.

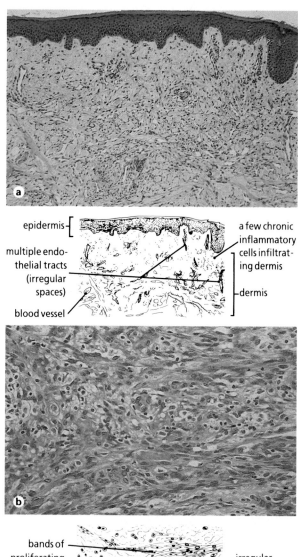

epidermis

a few chronic inflammatory cells infiltrating dermis

multiple endothelial tracts (irregular spaces)

dermis

blood vessel

bands of proliferating spindle cells

inflammatory cells

irregular channels with trapped red blood cells

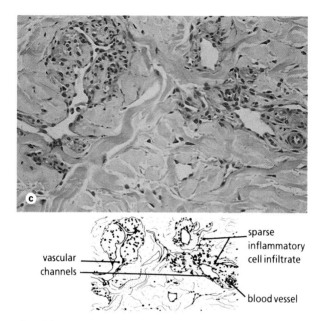

Fig. 67 (a) Low power view of Kaposi's sarcoma from a patient with AIDS. Numerous endothelial lined spaces are present throughout the dermis but spindle cells are not a prominent feature. **(b)** Medium power view of classical Kaposi's sarcoma. The tumour consists of bands of spindle cells with red blood cells in between. **(c)** Medium power view of a very early Kaposi's sarcoma lesion from a patient with AIDS. A few irregular vascular channels are surrounded by a sparse infiltrate of chronic inflammatory cells.

Lymphoma

The revision of the CDC Surveillance Definition of AIDS in 1987 took into account extracranial lymphoid neoplasia in HIV seropositive patients. Both Hodgkin's (Fig. 68) and, more often non-Hodgkin's lymphoma have been reported. Cerebral lymphoma (Fig. 69) and certain types of non-Hodgkin's lymphoma (NHL) are now diagnostic of AIDS.

In the majority of cases presentation of disease is late, at Stage III–IV. Extranodal (Fig. 70), especially CNS, gastrointestinal tract and bone marrow involvement, is common. A diagnosis of lymphoma should be considered in any patient presenting with weight loss, constitutional symptoms and anaemia.

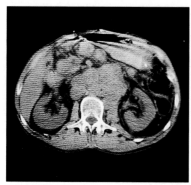

Fig.68 CT scan of the abdomen: there are large para-aortic lymph nodes. Biopsy confirmed a Hodgkin's lymphoma. Courtesy of Dr M Spittle.

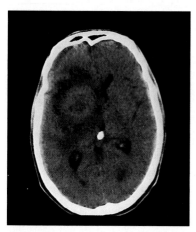

Fig.69 CT scan of the head: there is a large mass with ill defined borders in the left cerebral hemisphere. This was histologically confirmed as a cerebral lymphoma. The main differential diagnosis was cerebral toxoplasmosis. Courtesy of Professor S G Semple.

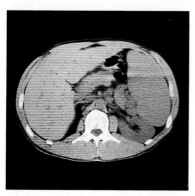

Fig.70 CT scan of the abdomen: there is marked hepatosplenomegaly. Biopsy confirmed a non-Hodgkin's lymphoma. Courtesy of Dr N Smith.

The clinical course is normally aggressive for both Hodgkin's and non-Hodgkin's lymphoma; patients with NHL rarely survive more than 5–6 months.

Histologically, nearly all NHL is high or intermediate grade, large or small cell, diffusively aggressive (Fig. 71) and of B cell immunophenotype. Similarly, the clinical course of Hodgkin's lymphoma is frequently atypical and aggressive.

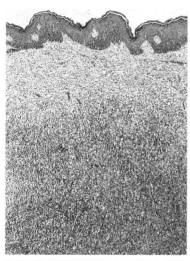
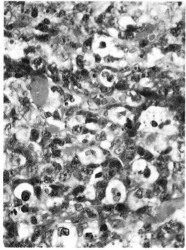

Fig.71 Low and high power views of a high grade malignant lymphoma infiltrating the skin. H & E stain. Courtesy of Dr N Smith.

Other Tumours

There are numerous reports of other tumours occurring in HIV seropositive patients, squamous cell carcinoma (Figs 72 & 73) at various sites being reported most often. There is, however, no epidemiological evidence of an increased incidence compared to the general population. Human papilloma virus infection may play a role in tumours of the oral cavity and anogenital tract.

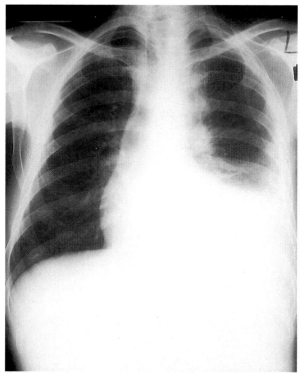

Fig.72 Chest X-ray. The left hilum is enlarged and there is a left pleural effusion. Bronchoscopy confirmed squamous cell carcinoma of the bronchus. Courtesy of Professor S G Semple.

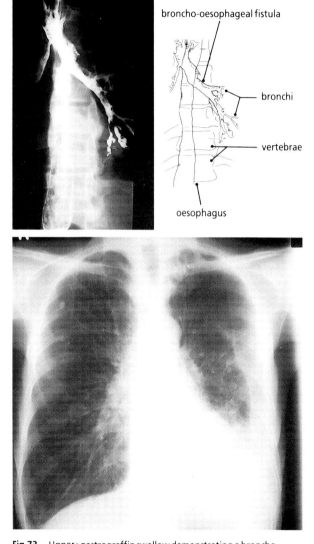

Fig. 73 Upper: gastrograffin swallow demonstrating a broncho-oesophageal fistula in a patient with a history of pneumocystis pneumonia nine months prior. Lower: chest X-ray of the same patient. There is a small left-sided pleural effusion and bronchogram following the swallow. Biopsy taken on endoscopy confirmed a squamous cell carcinoma of the bronchus. Courtesy of Professor S G Semple.

THE OPPORTUNISTIC INFECTIONS

Introduction

The opportunistic infections occurring in AIDS patients pose a host of formidable clinical problems. The organisms responsible are unusual pathogens; most of the infections are due to reactivation of latent organisms in the host or, in some cases, to ubiquitous organisms to which we are continually exposed. The infections are often difficult to diagnose because conventional serological tests are usually unhelpful. Treatment often suppresses rather than eradicates the organisms. Consequently relapses are common and continuous treatment with drugs, which may cause side effects, may be necessary.

Three main organ systems are affected – the respiratory system, the gastrointestinal tract, and the central nervous system. In addition, patients may present with a history of night sweats, chronic ill health, pyrexias or weight loss.

The pulmonary syndrome

CAUSES OF PULMONARY SYNDROME	
Bronchoscopy results from 102 patients with respiratory symptoms	(%)
Pneumocystis carinii pneumonia (PCP)	62.8
Cytomegalovirus	12.7
Kaposi's sarcoma	5.5
Lymphoid interstitial pneumonitis	2.7
Pneumococcus	3.7
PCP + atypical mycobacteria	0.9
TB + *Staph. aureus*	0.9
Staph. aureus	0.9
Actinomycosis	0.9
No diagnosis	9.0

Fig. 74 Causes of pulmonary syndrome. Bronchoscopy results from 102 patients with respiratory symptoms presenting to the Middlesex Hospital. Note that some patients have more than one diagnosis.

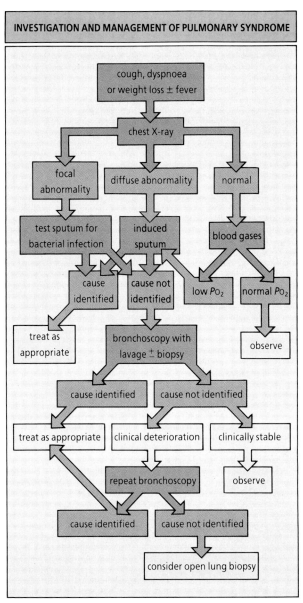

Fig. 75 Investigation and management of pulmonary syndrome.

CLINICAL FEATURES OF *PNEUMOCYSTIS CARINII* PNEUMONIA (PCP)	
Typical of PCP	**Not typical of PCP**
Recent onset of dyspnoea	
Dry cough ± mucoid sputum	Productive cough, purulent sputum
Inability to take a deep breath in	Chest pain (± pleuritic)
	Haemoptysis
Examination of chest: fine end inspiratory crackles (especially basally) or normal examination	Examination of chest: signs of consolidation or effusion
Chest x-ray: bilateral alveolar/ interstitial shadowing or normal	Chest x-ray: focal abnormalities e.g.: lobar, consolidation or pleural effusion(s) or mediastinal lymphadenopathy
Blood gases: hypoxaemia	

Fig. 76 Clinical features of *Pneumocystis carinii* pneumonia. If this occurs, the patient should initially be treated for PCP and if there is no response, another organism should be considered.

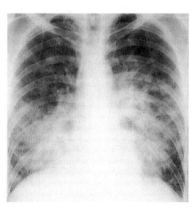

Fig. 77 Chest X-ray. Confluent opacities are present in both lung fields, especially in the lower zones. This is a typical feature of PCP, which is the most common life-threatening opportunistic infection in patients with AIDS.

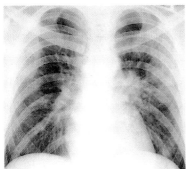

Fig. 78 Chest X-ray. Diffuse bilateral reticular infiltrates. *Pneumocystis carinii* was isolated from broncho-alveolar lavage specimens.

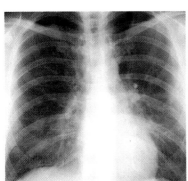

Fig. 79 In patients with early PCP the X-ray may be normal or show only minor changes. This X-ray shows minimal opacification in both lung fields, however *Pneumocystis carinii* was isolated from broncho-alveolar lavage specimens.

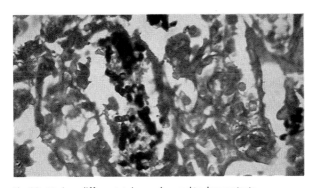

Fig. 80 Various different stains can be used to demonstrate *Pneumocystis carinii*. In this methenamine silver stain from a bronchoalveolar lavage, *Pneumocystis carinii* cysts are shown as densely staining clusters. Trophozoites may be demonstrated using a Giemsa stain. Courtesy of Professor H P Lambert.

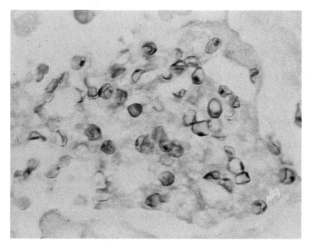

Fig. 81 Bronchial aspirate containing *Pneumocystis carinii* cysts. Grocott stain (methenamine silver counterstained with Malachite green), × 320.

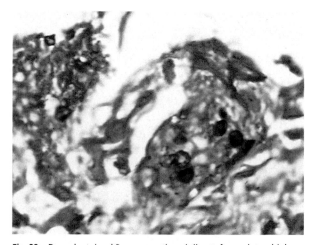

Fig. 82 Densely stained *Pneumocystis carinii* cysts from a bronchial aspirate. Methenamine silver counterstained with carbol fuchsin, × 320.

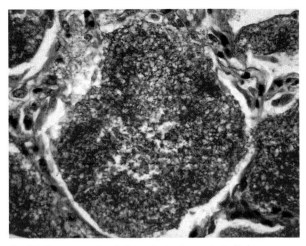

Fig. 83 *Pneumocystis carinii* may also be demonstrated in lung biopsies. This example shows a mass of organisms completely filling the alveolar spaces. H & E stain. Courtesy of Professor H P Lambert.

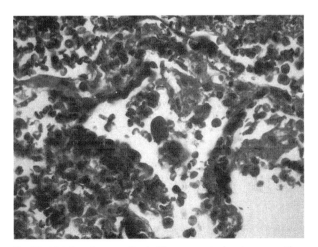

Fig. 84 Histology from a patient with pneumonia showing congestion and infiltration of the alveolar walls and an 'owl's eye' cell, typical of CMV, in the alveolar space. CMV is not uncommonly isolated from bronchial aspirate or biopsy in patients with AIDS, however the pathogenesis is often difficult to determine. Additional pathogens will be isolated from most patients. H & E stain. Courtesy of Professor H P Lambert.

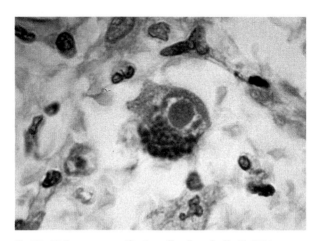

Fig. 85 High power magnification of 'owl's eye' cell with CMV inclusion. H & E stain. Courtesy of Professor H P Lambert.

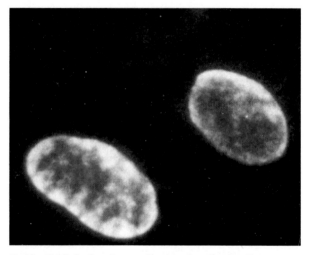

Fig. 86 CMV infection diagnosed by detection of early antigen-fluorescent foci (DEAFF). Monolayer cell cultures of human embryo lung fibroblasts were fixed after 24 hours' incubation and stained with monoclonal antibodies specific for CMV followed by fluorescein-conjugated goat anti-mouse IgG. Two fluorescent nuclei are seen. Early detection of CMV infection may help institute therapy with new antiviral drugs which are active against CMV. Courtesy of Dr P Griffiths; prepared by Mr P Stirk.

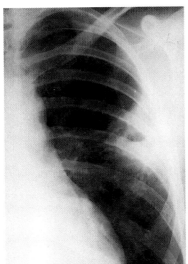

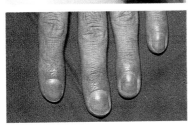

Fig. 87 Upper: chest X-ray of an HIV antibody-positive man with a lung abscess from which *Mycobacterium xenopi* was isolated. Atypical mycobacteria (especially *M. avium intracellulare)* are commonly isolated in AIDS patients. These organisms are often resistant to conventional antituberculosis therapy. Lower: the same patient later developed finger clubbing.

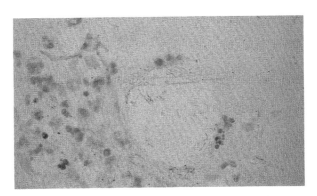

Fig. 88 Sputum specimen from a patient with a mycobacterial infection showing large numbers of typical acid-fast bacilli. Ziehl-Neelsen stain. Courtesy of Dr J F John, Jr.

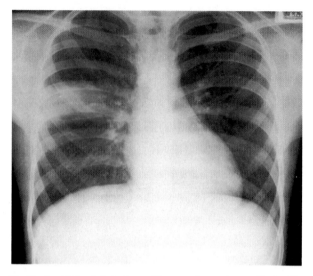

Fig. 89 In addition to infections with unusual organisms, patients with AIDS may develop bacterial pneumonia, the most common cause of which is *Streptococcus pneumoniae*. This X-ray of a patient with Kaposi's sarcoma shows a right upper lobe pneumonia. Pneumococci were isolated from the bronchial aspirate. Other bacteria which might be isolated include *Haemophilus influenzae*, Group B streptococci, *Branhamella catarrhalis*, and *Pseudomonas aeruginosa*.

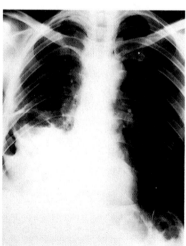

Fig. 90 X-ray of a lobulated empyema in an HIV antibody-positive patient with PGL. *Streptococcus pneumoniae* was isolated from the sputum.

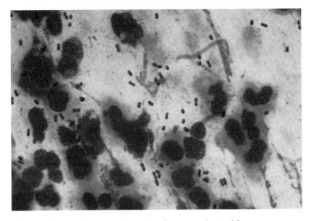

Fig. 91 Gram stained film of sputum from a patient with pneumococcal pneumonia showing characteristic lanceolate diplococci. Courtesy of Dr J R Contey.

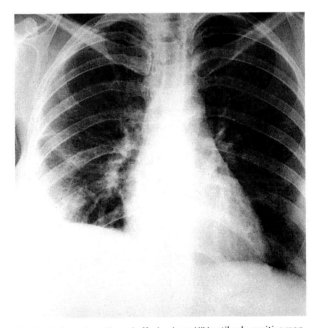

Fig. 92 Tuberculosis. Pleural effusion in an HIV antibody-positive man. Pulmonary tuberculosis may occur in HIV antibody-positive patients prior to the diagnosis of AIDS.

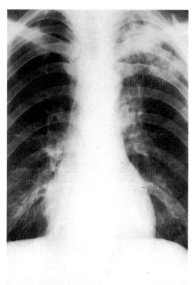

Fig. 93 Chest X-ray of an AIDS patient who presented with disseminated TB involving the lungs and the large bowel. Cavitating lesions can be seen in the left upper zone.

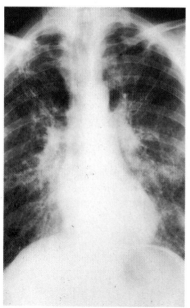

Fig. 94 Chest X-ray of a 32-year-old homosexual man who presented with dyspnoea. Perihilar infiltrates with areas of consolidation are visible in the left lower zone. *Pneumocystis carinii* pneumonia was diagnosed. The patient was still on antituberculosis treatment for pulmonary TB, diagnosed 10 months previously. Evidence of healing TB can be seen in the right upper zone.

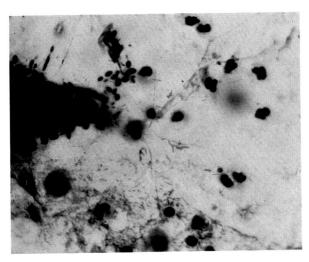

Fig. 95 Sputum from a patient with TB showing typical pink-staining mycobacteria. Ziehl-Neelsen stain, ×320.

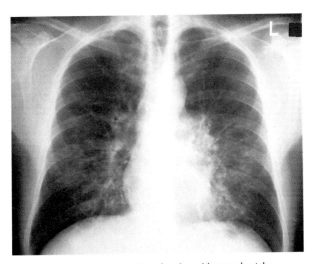

Fig. 96 Chest X-ray of AIDS patient showing widespread patchy shadowing in both lung fields. *Mycobacterium xenopi* was isolated from broncho-alveolar lavage specimens. Atypical mycobacterial lung infections are not uncommon but usually follow an indolent course, occur in the late stages of AIDS and may be an incidental finding. Treatment is difficult.

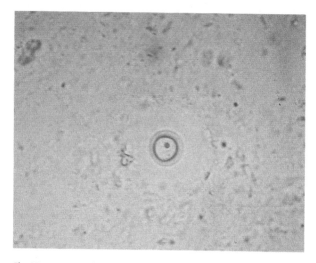

Fig. 97 An unusual organism, *Cryptococcus neoformans* is visible in this sputum specimen. The thick cell wall with a prominent vacuole and mucinous capsule are evident. KOH preparation. Courtesy of Dr A E Prevost.

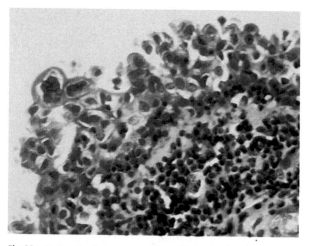

Fig. 98 Herpes simplex pneumonia lung biopsy showing subepithelial proliferation of mononuclear cells and a single inclusion body in an epithelial cell. This virus is a rare cause of pneumonia but is important to diagnose because effective treatment is available. Courtesy of Professor H P Lambert.

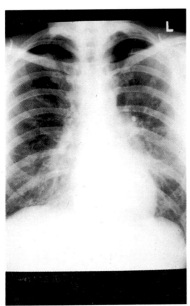

Fig. 99 Kaposi's sarcoma may cause lung infiltrates which, using conventional radiology, are indistinguishable from those in *Pneumocystis carinii* pneumonia. This patient with extensive Kaposi's sarcoma has infiltrates in both lung fields. Bronchoalveolar lavage revealed no organisms, however extensive Kaposi's sarcoma was seen on bronchoscopy and confirmed on biopsy.

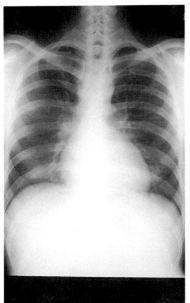

Fig. 100 Interstitial pneumonitis. Chronic lymphoid interstitial pneumonitis is a major presenting complaint in children with AIDS. The chest X-ray shows bilateral reticulonodular interstitial infiltrates, which may be indistinguishable from PCP. Biopsy reveals a diffuse nodular lymphocytic infiltrate.

The CNS syndrome

NEUROLOGICAL COMPLICATIONS IN 186 PATIENTS WITH HIV INFECTION	
Central Nervous System	**number (%)**
Viral infections	
AIDS-related dementia	30 (16)
CMV encephalitis	3 (2)
CMV retinitis	9 (5)
HIV-related meningitis	13 (17)
Progressive multifocal leukoencephalopathy	1 (0.5)
Intracranial mass lesions	
Cerebral toxoplasmosis	15 (8)
Primary CNS lymphoma	7 (4)
Undefined mass lesions	6 (3)
Systemic lymphoma	1 (0.5)
Peripheral Nervous System	**number (%)**
Inflammatory demyelinating neuropathy	11 (6)
Sensory neuropathy	26 (14)
Cranial neuropathies	4 (2)
Multiple mononeuropathies	2 (1)
Herpes zoster myeloradiculitis	8 (4)
Miscellaneous	**number (%)**
Cryptococcal meningitis	11 (6)
Neurosyphilis (treated)	1 (0.5)
Metabolic encephalopathy	5 (3)
Cerebrovascular accident	1 (0.5)

Fig. 101 Neurological complications of AIDS. Modified from McArthur et al. (1987) *Medicine* **66** : 407-437.

DIAGNOSTIC FEATURES OF AIDS-RELATED DEMENTIA (HIV ENCEPHALOPATHY)

Mandatory

Positive HIV serology

History of cognitive/behavioural changes
    memory loss, apathy, impaired concentration & attention

Neurological findings
    hyperreflexia, hypertonia, release signs, myelopathy

CT/MRI
    atrophy, changes in white matter

CSF
    ↑ IgG & total protein, normal cell count, negative
    cryptococcal antigen & syphilis serology

Exclude
    cryptococcal meningitis, metabolic/drug encephalopathy,
    intracranial mass lesion, neurosyphilis

Optional

Detailed neuropsychological testing

CSF
    HIV isolation, p24 antigen, intrathecal synthesis of HIV
    specific antibodies

Brain biopsy/autopsy
    multinucleated giant cells, microglial nodules, HIV
    isolation/in situ hybridization/immunostaining

Fig. 102 Diagnostic features of AIDS-related dementia (HIV encephalopathy).

CLINICAL FEATURES OF OTHER NEUROLOGICAL SYNDROMES ASSOCIATED WITH HIV INFECTION

Condition	Clinical features
Vacuolar myelopathy	bi- or unilateral leg weakness paraesthesia or sensory loss ataxia incontinence
Aseptic meningitis	headaches fever meningeal irritation cranial nerve palsies
Polyneuropathy	inflammatory demyelinating acute (Guillain–Barré syndrome) or chronic sensorimotor

Fig. 103 Clinical features of other neurological syndromes associated with HIV infection.

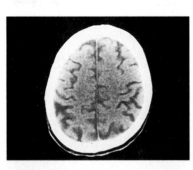

Fig. 104 HIV encephalopathy. CT scan showing prominent cortical sulci indicative of cerebral atrophy.

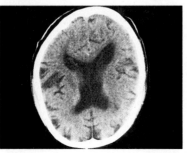

Fig. 105 HIV encephalopathy. CT scan showing dilated ventricles.

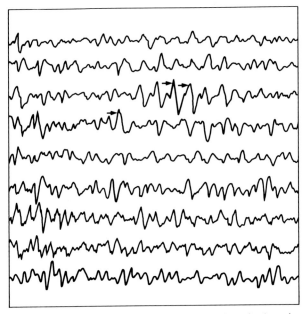

Fig. 106 HIV encephalopathy. Severely disorganized EEG dominated by regular slow activity (arrowed). Courtesy of Dr M Harrison.

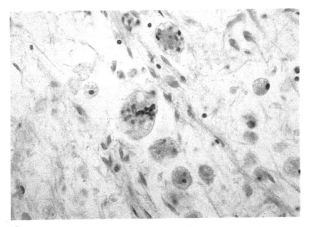

Fig. 107 H & E stain of brain tissue obtained at post-mortem from a man with HIV encephalopathy showing collection of macrophages and typical multinucleated giant cells. Courtesy of Dr F Scaravilli, Institute of Neurology.

DIFFERENTIAL DIAGNOSIS OF HIV ENCEPHALOPATHY

Cerebral toxoplasmosis

CMV encephalitis

CNS lymphoma

Cryptococcal meningitis

Metabolic disorders

Psychiatric conditions

Drugs

Fig. 108 Differential diagnosis of HIV encephalopathy.

CLINICAL FEATURES OF CEREBRAL TOXOPLASMOSIS

lethargy

confusion

focal neurological signs & symptoms

altered levels of consciousness

seizures

Fig. 109 Clinical features of cerebral toxoplasmosis.

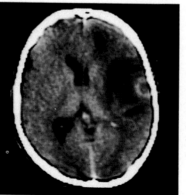

Fig. 110 Contrast enhanced CT scan from a man with cerebral toxoplasmosis showing a ring enhancing lesion with surrounding cerebral oedema. Similar lesions have been reported in AIDS patients with cerebral candidiasis, tuberculosis, lymphomas or CMV infections.

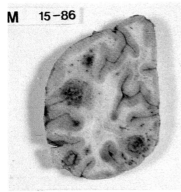

Fig. 111 Post-mortem specimen showing multiple lesions in an HIV-positive drug abuser; these were due to cerebral toxoplasmosis. Courtesy of Dr F Scaravilli.

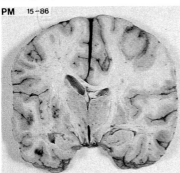

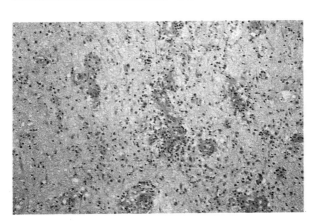

Fig. 112 Marked perivascular inflammation in a patient with cerebral toxoplasmosis. H & E stain, × 40. Courtesy of Dr F Scaravilli.

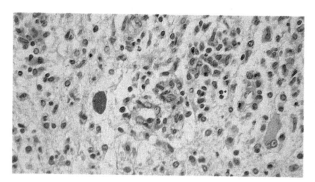

Fig. 113 Toxoplasma cyst in a patient with cerebral toxoplasmosis. H & E stain. Courtesy of Dr F Scaravilli.

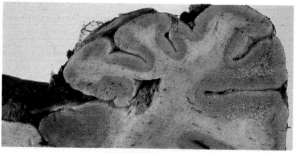

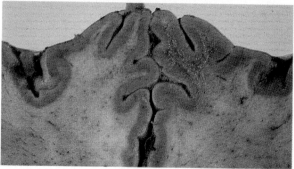

Fig. 114 Progressive multifocal leukoencephalopathy (PML) is a demyelinating disease probably caused by a papovavirus. Patients present with mental aberrations, aphasias, hemiparesis, ataxia, blindness and other focal signs. The outlook is grim with a steady decline until death. This post-mortem specimen shows PML with focal areas of demyelination. Courtesy of Dr F Scaravilli.

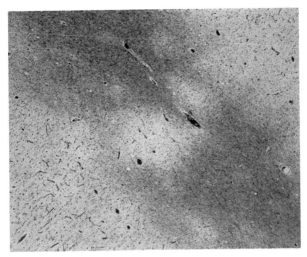

Fig. 115 Histological specimen from an HIV-positive male with PML. The demyelinated areas show up as pale blue. Luxol fast blue stain, × 10. Courtesy of Dr F Scaravilli.

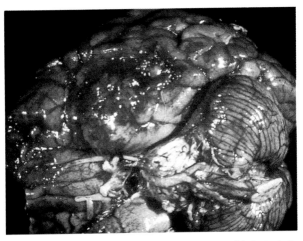

Fig. 116 HSV encephalitis. AIDS patients may present with the typical features of HSV encephalitis including seizures, hemiparesis or dysphasia. The virus has a prediliction for the frontal, temporal and parietal lobes. This gross specimen shows necrosis, haemorrhage and oedema involving the left frontal and temporal lobes. Courtesy of Professor H P Lambert.

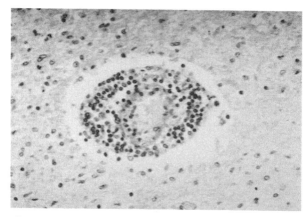

Fig. 117 Histological specimen from a patient with HSV encephalitis, showing a perivascular mononuclear inflammatory exudate with slight gliosis and inflammation in the grey matter of the temporal lobes. Occasionally, HSV is isolated from the brain of HIV antibody-positive patients who do not have typical HIV encephalitis. The significance of these isolates is not known. Courtesy of Professor H P Lambert.

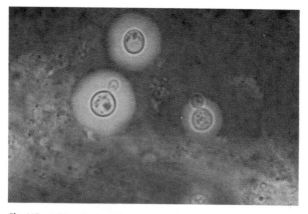

Fig. 118 AIDS patients with cryptococcal meningitis may present with headache, seizures and confusion; some may present with atypical features, presumably due to the minimal inflammatory response seen in immunocompromised patients. *Cryptococcus neoformans* is easily detected using an India ink preparation from CSF sediment. The internal structure of the yeast may be seen and the cell wall identified as a refractile structure. Cryptococcal antigen may be detected in the CSF. Courtesy of Dr A E Prevost.

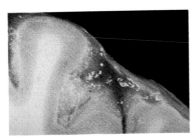

Fig. 119 Cryptococcal meningitis. Cross section of the frontal cortex showing gelatinous material in the sulci from the capsule of the organism. Courtesy of Professor H P Lambert.

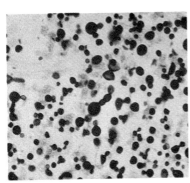

Fig. 120 *Cryptococcus neoformans* in exudate within the subarachnoid space. The capsule does not take up the methenamine silver stain. The microorganism may be detected by measuring cryptococcal antigen in the CSF. Courtesy of Professor H P Lambert.

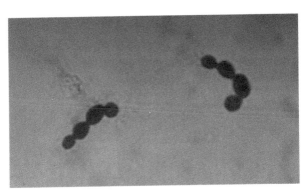

Fig. 121 Candidiasis is a rare infection of the CNS in patients with AIDS. It often presents with a single brain abscess and focal neurological signs, although meningoencephalitis and multiple microabscesses have been reported. Patients usually have evidence of *Candida albicans* infection elsewhere. The CSF may show typical candidal spores. Courtesy of Dr A E Prevost.

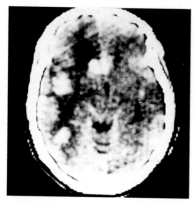

Fig. 122 CT scan showing multiple lesions. At post-mortem, these were found to be due to tuberculosis.

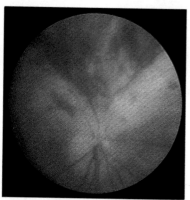

Fig. 123 Cytomegalovirus retinitis in a patient with AIDS. Extensive exudates and haemorrhages are visible. Without treatment there is a rapid decline in visual acuity and often ultimate blindness.

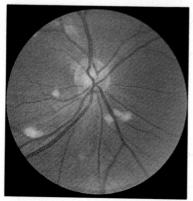

Fig. 124 Soft exudates also occur in HIV-positive patients. The pathogenesis of this condition is unknown.

The gut syndrome

CONDITIONS AFFECTING THE GASTROINTESTINAL TRACT AND LIVER IN AIDS	
Syndrome	**Causes**
Retrosternal discomfort/ dysphagia	Candidiasis Cytomegalovirus (CMV) Herpes simplex virus (HSV)
Diarrhoea/weight loss/ malabsorption	Unknown – enteropathy Cryptosporidium, *Isospora belli* and microsporidia CMV/HSV Mycobacteria Enteric bacteria – salmonella, campylobacter Neoplasia
Hepatitis/cholestasis	Mycobacteria Cryptosporidium CMV *Cryptococcus neoformans* Drug induced
Perianal ulceration	HSV ?CMV
Neoplasia and miscellaneous	Kaposi's sarcoma Lymphoma Hairy leukoplakia Recalcitrant anorectal warts ? Squamous oral/anal carcinoma

Fig. 125 Gastrointestinal complications of AIDS.

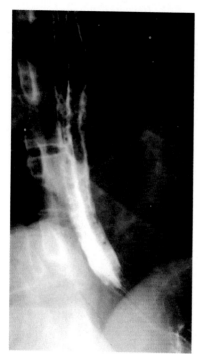

Fig. 126 Barium swallow in an HIV antibody-positive patient with dysphagia. The barium reveals multiple superficial plaques, or ulcers. The most common cause of this appearance is candidiasis; HSV and CMV infection are other possible causes, and may be radiologically indistinguishable from candidal infection. Upper gastrointestinal tract endoscopy with biopsy and culture is the only means of confirming the diagnosis.

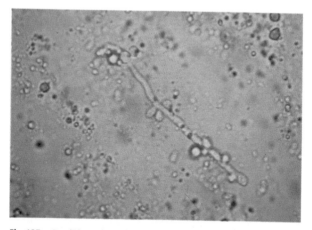

Fig. 127 *Candida* can be quickly and easily identified using a simple KOH preparation, in which the hyphae and yeast forms are easily seen. Courtesy of Dr A E Prevost.

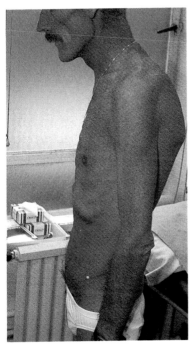

Fig. 128 Chronic diarrhoea can result in prolonged debility and wasting, as seen here. Often no cause can be found.

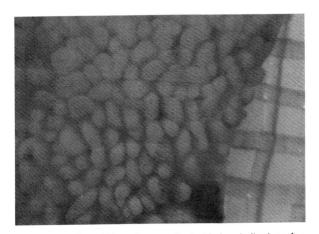

Fig. 129 Small bowel biopsy from a patient with chronic diarrhoea for which no cause could be found. The biopsy shows partial villous atrophy with broadened and flattened villi. This may be due to HIV itself. ×20

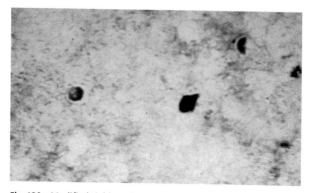

Fig. 130 Modified Ziehl-Neelsen stain showing Cryptosporidium. This is the most common organism identified in AIDS patients with diarrhoea. The diarrhoea is often profuse and watery.

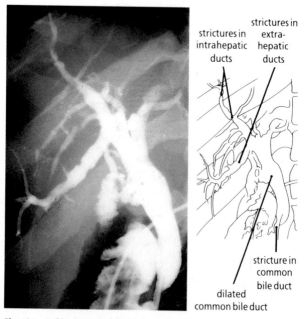

strictures in intrahepatic ducts

strictures in extra-hepatic ducts

stricture in common bile duct

dilated common bile duct

Fig. 131 A dilated common bile duct and intrahepatic ducts can be seen on endoscopic retrograde cholangiopancreatography in patients with cryptosporidial or CMV infection of the biliary tree. Patients may present with abdominal pain, fever and a raised alkaline phosphatase level.

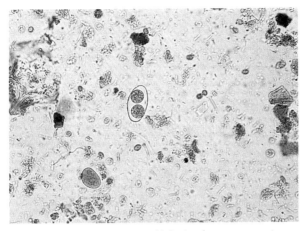

Fig. 132 *Isospora belli* is a protozoal infection that can cause watery diarrhoea in AIDS patients; it is indistinguisable from that caused by Cryptosporidium. This unstained concentrated stool specimen shows an oocyst of *Isospora belli* with two sporoblasts.

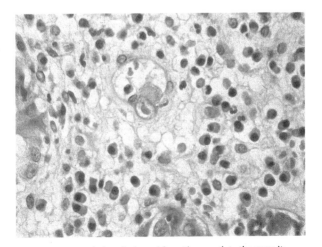

Fig. 133 CMV can infect the bowel from the mouth to the anus. It usually causes ulceration but has been associated with diarrhoea, abdominal pain and involvement of the biliary tree. This biopsy was taken from a patient with diarrhoea and shows an inflammatory infiltrate and an 'owl's eye' inclusion, typical of CMV. Although CMV can be isolated and typical inclusions seen in biopsies, the role of the virus in pathogenesis remains unproven.

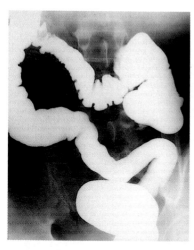

Fig. 134 TB of the bowel in an HIV antibody-positive patient. This barium enema shows an oedematous, rather featureless terminal ileum. Although therapy is often successful in these cases, other opportunistic infections often complicate the clinical picture and response.

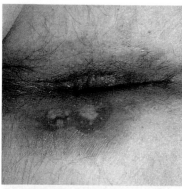

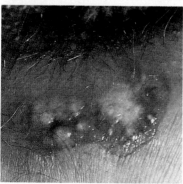

Fig. 135 Severe perianal herpes simplex virus (HSV) infection. This may be the presenting complaint in patients with AIDS. The ulcers often occur intermittently, but eventually they are persistent and involve increasingly larger areas of skin and mucous membranes. Upper: this patient presented with a well circumscribed area of ulceration. Lower: a closer view of the ulceration shows marked erythema and a haemorrhagic base.

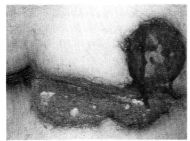

Fig. 136 Large area of perianal ulceration due to HSV.

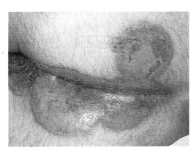

Fig. 137 The same patient showing complete epithelialization 10 days after commencing treatment with intravenous acyclovir.

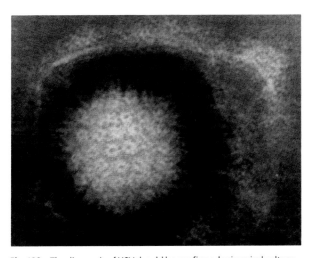

Fig. 138 The diagnosis of HSV should be confirmed using viral culture. Electronmicroscopy (EM), using a scraping from a lesion, is a more rapid technique. This illustration shows a typical herpes group virus, however, this technique does not differentiate between HSV, CMV, varicella-zoster and Epstein-Barr virus. Courtesy of the Welcomme Institute.

TREATMENT OF PROTOZOAL OPPORTUNISTIC INFECTIONS

Infection	Drug	Duration	Side effects	Comments
Pneumocystis carinii pneumonia treatment	cotrimoxazole (trimethoprim 20mg/kg/day), iv × 14 days then oral	14–21 days	nausea fever rash marrow suppression	80% of patients will respond to treatment.
	or			
	pentamidine isethionate (4mg/kg) day	14–21 days	hypotension hypoglycaemia renal failure hepatitis marrow suppression	
	or			
	pentamidine mesylate (2.5mg/kg) day – both as a slow iv infusion			
	or			
	nebulized pentamidine isethionate (8mg/kg) day	14–21 days	bronchospasm metallic taste	Patients may prefer as no iv therapy + fewer side effects.

Fig. 139 Treatment of protozoal opportunistic infections.

Pneumocystis carinii pneumonia maintenance	cotrimoxazole 960mg daily or alternate days or Fansidar 1 tablet weekly or dapsone 100mg weekly or inhaled pentamidine 8mg/kg every 2–4 weeks	indefinite	usually minimal	Exact dose or frequency not yet established.
Toxoplasmosis	pyremethamine 25mg daily oral + sulphadiazine 2–4mg daily po or clindamycin 500mg qds po	indefinite indefinite	rash nausea marrow suppression	May be possible to reduce frequency and dose during maintenance.
Cryptosporidium	spiramycin 1gm qds or erythromycin 500mg qds or clindamycin 300mg qds and quinine 250mg qds	14 days 14 days 14 days	nausea rashes	No treatment is of proven value.
Isosporiasis	cotrimoxazole 2 tabs qds oral	indefinite	see above	

TREATMENT OF VIRAL OPPORTUNISTIC INFECTIONS

Infection	Drug	Duration	Side effects	Comments
Herpes simplex treatment	acyclovir 200mg 5 × daily po or 5–10mg/kg 8 hourly iv	10–14 days		
prophylaxis	acyclovir 200mg qds	indefinite		May be possible to reduce frequency.
Cytomegalovirus treatment	ganciclovir 5mg/kg bd	14–21 days	anaemia neutropenia	Marrow suppression potentiated with zidovudine.
prophylaxis	ganciclovir (2.5–5.0mg/kg) day	indefinite	anaemia neutropenia	

Fig. 140 Treatment of viral opportunistic infections.

TREATMENT OF FUNGAL OPPORTUNISTIC INFECTIONS

Infection	Drug	Duration	Side effects	Comments
Candidiasis local treatment	nystatin oral suspension, or pastilles, miconazole oral gel, amphotericin lozenges – all 4–6 × daily	PRN		Relapse common, many patients require systemic therapy.
systemic treatment	ketoconazole 200–400mg oral daily	indefinite	nausea hepatitis thrombocytopenia	Relapse common on cessation of treatment.
maintenance	fluconazole 200–400mg daily 100mg fluconazole daily	6 weeks indefinite	nausea	Relapse may occur, maintenance needed.
Cryptococcosis	amphotericin B (0.3mg/kg) day + flucytosine (150mg/kg) day in 4 doses	5 weeks	nausea, vomiting, rashes, bone marrow suppression, renal damage, hypocalcaemia	
	fluconazole 200–400mg daily	6 weeks	nausea	

Fig. 141 Treatment of fungal opportunistic infections.

ANTIVIRAL AGENTS AND VACCINES

Antiviral agents

The high morbidity and mortality associated with HIV infection has made the development of an effective antiviral agent a high priority for medical research. Current developments aim at:

- Interrupting the replication cycle of HIV (Fig. 142). There are many possible targets for intervention by anti-HIV agents (Fig. 143), but the qualities of the ideal agent (Fig. 144) are difficult to satisfy.

- Providing supportive immunotherapy (Fig. 145).

Future developments may involve both.

The viral enzyme reverse transcriptase catalyses the formation of a DNA copy of the viral RNA genome. Inhibition of this enzyme and the subsequent termination of the developing DNA chain has proved the most successful strategy so far. Dideoxynucleoside analogues are a group of drugs which act in this way. Of these, zidovudine is the only one to date which has been used extensively in the treatment of patients with AIDS and ARC.

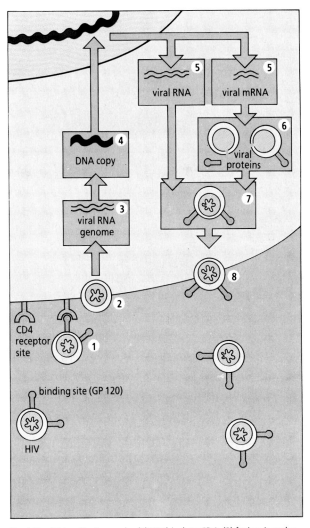

Fig. 142 HIV replication cycle: (1) HIV binds to CD4; (2) fusion (may be by endocytosis) followed by release of viral RNA into cell cytoplasm; (3) transcription of viral RNA genome by reverse transcriptase to DNA copy; (4) integration; (5) transcription of DNA copy to viral RNA and viral messenger RNA; (6) translation of mRNA to viral proteins; (7) viral product assembly; (8) budding of intact virion. The CD4$^+$ cell may be a T helper lymphocyte, a B lymphocyte, a monocyte/macrophage, a dendritic cell or a microglial cell.

ANTI-HIV AGENTS	
Target	**Agent**
HIV binding to target cell	soluble CD4 peptides, dextran sulphate, monoclonal antibodies, anti-idiotype antibodies
reverse transcriptase	dideoxynucleoside analogues (zidovudine, dideoxycytidine and others in development), phosphonoformate, rifamycin derivatives e.g. ansamycin
integration of virus	viral integrase inhibitors
transcription of viral genome	RNA polymerase inhibitors
translation of viral mRNA	inhibitors e.g. ribavirin oligonucleotides (anti-sense constructs) viral regulatory gene inhibitors
viral product assembly & modification	glycosylation inhibitors, e.g. glucosidase inhibitors, protein kinase inhibitors, viral protease inhibitors
viral budding	inhibitors e.g. interferons (also act at other sites)

Fig. 143 Anti-HIV agents. Combinations of agents acting at different sites may be synergistic and allow lower doses, thus reducing the overall toxicity.

IDEAL ANTI-HIV AGENT

Low toxicity

High specificity for HIV and
HIV infected cells

Protects uninfected cells

Penetrates CSF

Orally absorbed

Long half-life

Produced at low cost

Fig. 144 Properties of the ideal anti-HIV agent.

IMMUNOTHERAPY FOR HIV INFECTION

Lymphokines
γ-interferon
α-interferon (synergistic with zidovudine)
interleukin-2
tumour necrosis factor
lymphokine inducers e.g. mismatched double-stranded
RNA polymers

Human granulocyte colony stimulating factor
(? reverses HIV related leucopenia)

Bone marrow transplantation & antiviral therapy

Passive immunization e.g. anti-P24 antibodies

Active immunization (vaccine) may protect against
disease progression

Fig. 145 Immunotherapy for HIV infection.

Zidovudine

Substitution of a hydroxyl group in the 3′ position in the nucleoside thymidine by an azido group forms the dideoxynucleoside analogue zidovudine (Fig. 146). Following phosphorylation, thymidine is able to form a 3′–5′ phosphodiester bond in the developing DNA chain. Alternatively, if zidovudine is incorporated, the DNA chain is effectively terminated as the presence of the azido group prevents the formation of further phosphodiester bonds. *In vitro* testing has shown that zidovudine has a higher affinity for HIV polymerase (reverse transcriptase) than for other cellular DNA polymerases, but inhibition of DNA synthesis in actively dividing host cells accounts for the main toxic side effect of the drug – bone marrow suppression (Fig. 147).

Clinical trials have shown that the use of zidovudine extends the life expectancy of patients with ARC and AIDS (Fig. 148), however, long-term tolerance of the drug is low, with 50% of patients needing to stop therapy at one time or other.

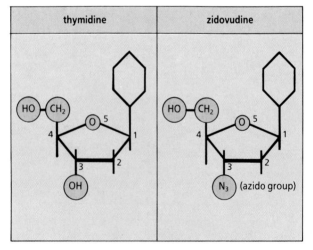

Fig. 146 Substitution of a hydroxyl group in the 3′ position in the nucleoside thymidine (left) by an azido group forms the dideoxynucleoside analogue zidovudine (right). Incorporation of the latter into a developing DNA chain causes termination, as the azido group prevents formation of further phosphodiester bonds.

SIDE EFFECTS OF ZIDOVUDINE

general

Gastrointestinal
  nausea ⎫
  vomiting ⎬ common

Insomnia (common)
  myalgia
  headaches

Myopathy after long-term therapy

haematological

Peripheral blood:
  red blood cell — macrocytosis,
                  anaemia
  white blood cell — leucopenia,
                  neutropenia
  platelets — thrombocytopenia

Bone marrow:
  megaloblastic change
  pure erythroid hypoplasia

Fig. 147 Side effects of zidovudine.

EFFICACY OF ZIDOVUDINE

↓ mortality

↓ incidence & severity of opportunistic
  infection

↓ constitutional symptoms

↑ CD4$^+$ count (significant but modest
  and transient)

↓ P24 (approximately 90% reduction)

Fig. 148 Efficacy of zidovudine.

Haematological Toxicity

Over 50% of patients with ARC and AIDS will experience haematological toxicity in the form of one or more cytopenias. These are reversible with cessation of therapy. With regular full blood count monitoring complications of severe toxicity should be avoided by blood transfusion, dose modification or interruption.

Examination of the bone marrow reveals a variety of changes, including variable cellularity, megaloblastic changes and erythroid dysplasias (Figs 149–151).

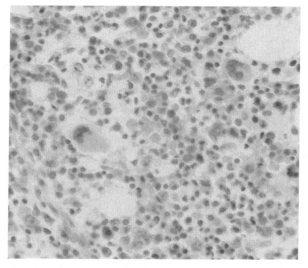

Fig. 149 Bone marrow trephine biopsy showing red cell hypoplasia. There is general hyperplasia but erythroid precursors are absent. This patient developed marked anaemia after 8 weeks on zidovudine. ×400. Courtesy of Dr H Cohen and Dr F Matthey.

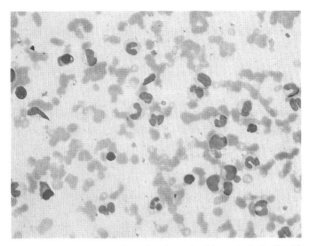

Fig. 150 Bone marrow aspirate showing red cell hypoplasia. Erythroid precursors are absent. This patient had been receiving long-term zidovudine treatment and needed recurrent blood transfusions, ×250. Courtesy of Dr H Cohen and Dr F Matthey.

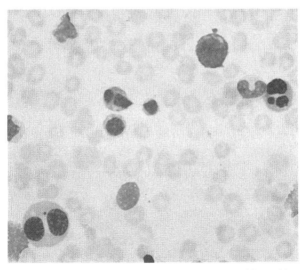

Fig. 151 Bone marrow aspirate showing dysplastic normoblasts. This patient developed a severe pancytopenia after 3 months' treatment with zidovudine, ×400. Courtesy of Dr H Cohen and Dr F Matthey.

Vaccines

The development of an effective vaccine against HIV has encountered many problems (Fig. 152). Traditionally, the whole virus in an attenuated or killed form is used to stimulate a primary immune response which is protective. Presentation of HIV in this way is widely felt to be unsafe because of the possibility of infection. Rapid mutation of HIV may lead to reversion to full potency.

PROBLEMS WITH HIV VACCINE DEVELOPMENT	
Whole virus vaccines	
live attenuated or killed	Risk of infection — ? unsafe
Subunit vaccines	
Antigens	Envelope proteins — high frequency of genetic mutation; vaccines may be active against only some viral strains (but conserved epitopes exist)
	Core proteins — ? promote cell mediated immune response
Manufacture	Viral culture — difficult Synthetic peptides Recombinant gene techniques (yeast, mammalian, bacterial, insect cells)
Efficacy	Neutralizing antibodies — ? protective Viral antigens — ? immunosuppressive ? Role of cell mediated immune response
Evaluation	Absence of ideal animal model for testing Human trials

Fig. 152   Problems with HIV vaccine development.

Two main approaches have been used to overcome this problem. The first involves the use of parts or subunits of the HIV envelope and the second uses CD4 antibodies (anti-idiotype) as the vaccine antigen. Subunit antigens can be derived from virus cultures, manufactured synthetically or genetically engineered. Most of the candidate vaccines are based on outer envelope proteins. Presentation of these subunit viral antigens may or may not stimulate production of neutralizing antibodies in a high enough titre to be protective. A variety of techniques and adjuvants have been developed to enhance the immune response (Fig. 153). Some subunit vaccines are undergoing preliminary trials in human volunteers.

In the anti-idiotype approach, antibodies (idiotype) are raised against $CD4^+$ cell receptor sites and these are used as a vaccine antigen to promote production of antibodies (anti-idiotype) which are the mirror-image of the $CD4^+$ cell receptor site. These anti-idiotype antibodies can bind to the receptor site on the viral envelope, thus preventing the virus from infecting $CD4^+$ cells (Fig. 154).

Whichever vaccine is used, evaluation in human trials (Fig. 155) will be difficult.

TECHNIQUES TO ENHANCE THE IMMUNE RESPONSE TO VACCINE ANTIGENS

Conventional adjuvants
 e.g. aluminium salts

Novel antigen presentation
 immunostimulatory complexes (ISCOMS)
 liposomes
 yeast proteins ('pseudoviruses')
 monokines – lymphokines
 virus vectors (e.g. vaccinia) for HIV genes

Fig. 153 Techniques to enhance the immune response to vaccine antigen.

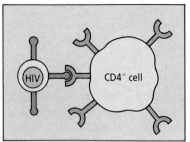

Fig. 154 Anti-idiotype vaccine. Antibodies are raised against CD4$^+$ receptors. These anti-CD4 antibodies are used as the vaccine antigen, stimulating production of anti-idiotype antibodies, which bind to GP120, blocking the HIV receptor site.

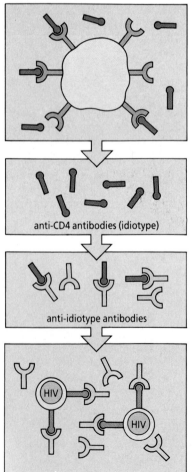

HUMAN VACCINE TRIALS		
	objective	no. of recipients
Phase I Phase II Phase III	safety & immunogenicity safety & immunogenicity efficacy	10 – 20 40 – 60 ?
Problems		

Ethical — information on primary prevention (e.g. safe sexual practices) must also be given to vaccine recipients

Vaccine recipients — ? target 'high risk' groups but:

1) changing sexual behaviour in developed world has already decreased new infection rate

2) recruitment & compliance problems (e.g. in IV drug abusers)

Fig. 155 Human vaccine trials.

INDEX

Abscesses
  brain 83
  dental 28
Acneform eruption 29
Actinomycosis 60
Acyclovir 33, 91, 94
AIDS-related
  complex (ARC) 27, 38, 40, 96, 102
  retrovirus phosphatase level raised 88
Amphotericin 95
Anaemia 38, 42, 55, 94, 102
Aphasias 80
Aphthous ulcer 28, 37
  mouth 36

Bacteria
  enteric 85
Bacterial
  infection 61
  infections 28
  pneumonia 68
Blindness 80
Bone marrow
  aspirate 40, 103
  trephine biopsy 38–39, 102
Brain biopsy/autopsy 75, 77, 79, 83
Branhamella catarrhalis 68
Bronchospasm 92

Campylobacter 85
Cancers
  secondary 23
Candida albicans 83
Candidiasis 83, 85–86
  cerebral 78
  interdigital 28
  oesophageal 2, 3
  oral 23, 37, 42
    severe 36
  perianal 28
  productive 62
  treatment 95

Carcinoma
  squamous cell 58–59
  squamous oral/anal 85
CD4 7
  peptides 98
  tropism 1
CD4$^+$ 8–11
  cell count
    fall in 38, 41
    increase in 101
  receptor 22
  tropism 19
CDC classification 23, 27, 55
Chemotherapy 53
Children, with AIDS 73
Clindamycin 93
CNS syndrome 74–84
Coccidioidomycosis
  disseminated 3
Confusion 78, 82
Constitutional
  disease 23
  symptoms 42, 55
  syndromes 27
Cotrimoxazole 92–93
Cough 61
Cryptococcosis
  extrapulmonary 2
  treatment 95
Cryptococcus neoformans 72, 82–83, 85
Cryptosporidial infection 88
Cryptosporidiosis 2
Cryptosporidium 85, 88–89
  treatment 93
Cytomegalovirus (CMV) 60, 65–66, 85, 89, 91
  encephalitis 74, 78
  infection 78, 88
  prophylaxis 94
  retinitis 3, 74, 84
  treatment 94
Cytopenia 102

Cytotoxic
  response 7
  T-cells 8
Cytotoxicity
  antibody-dependant cell
    (ADCC) 8

Dapsone 93
Definition
  of AIDS 2
Dental
  disease 28
Dementia 23, 74
  diagnostic features 75
Dermatofibromata 44
Dermatophyte infections 30
  chronic 33
Dideoxycytidine 98
Dysphasia 81, 86
Dysplasia
  erythroid 38, 102
  myeloid 38

Ecchymoses 44
Empyema
  lobulated 68
Encephalitis 25
  acute 24
  CMV 74, 78
  HSV 81–82
Encephalopathy
  CMV 78
  HIV 3, 75–78, 82
  metabolic 74, 75
Epstein–Barr virus 37, 91
ESR 42
Exanthema
  of acute infection 24

Fansidar 93
Fatigue 27
Fever 61, 76, 88, 92
Fevers 24, 27
Fluconazole 95
Flucytosine 95
Folliculitis 28
  diffuse 29

Fungal infection 32, 33, 38
Fungi 28

Ganciclovir 94
Genetic structure
  HIV 20
Genomic diversity
  of HIV 20
Gingivitis
  necrotizing ulcerative 28, 37
Gonorrhea rate 18
Granulocyte colony
  stimulating factor 99
Granuloma
  non-caseating 39
Gut syndrome 85

Hairy leukoplakia 28, 85
  oral 23, 37, 42
Headaches 76, 82, 101
Hepatitis 85, 92, 95
Hepatosplenomegaly 27, 56
Hemiparesis 80–81
Herpes simplex 2
  anogenital 28
  fauces 32
  genital 31
  labial 32
  palate 32
  perianal 31, 90, 91
  pneumonia 72
  prophylaxis 94
  treatment 94
Herpes zoster 23, 33
  myeloradiculitis 74
Heterosexual
  patient groups, USA 4
Histoplasmosis
  disseminated 3
Hilar nodes
  enlarged 27
Homosexual/bisexual men
  patient groups USA 4
  STD clinics, USA and UK
    17–18
  Kaposi's sarcoma 43
HTLV 10

HTLV–I 10, 20
HTLV–I I 10, 20
HTLV–I I I 10
HTLV–IV 20
Hyperplasia 102
Hyperreflexia 15
Hypertonia 75
Hypoglycaemia 92, 95
Hypoplasia
  erythroid 101
Hypotension 92

Immune dysfunction
  spectrum of 7
Immunization 1
Immunofluorescence
  fixed cell direct 12
Immunotherapy 99
Impetigo 28
Incontinence 76
α-interferon 53, 98
Interferon γ 8, 98
Interferons 98
Interleukin–1 8
Interleukin–2 98
Insomnia 101
Intravenous drug abusers
  patient groups, USA 4
Isospora belli 85, 89
Isosporiasis 3
  treatment 93
Inspiratory crackles
  fine end 62

Kaposi's sarcoma 27, 60, 68, 73
  aggressive form 1
  colon 43, 50
  duodenum 43
  gums 53
  gut syndrome 85
  histology 53–55
  indicative of HIV 2
  lesion
    disseminated 46–47
    early 44, 53
    later 44, 45
    nodular 43, 45
  polypoid 43
    telangiectatic 43
  lymphatic involvement
    48–49
  lymph node involvement
    43, 49
  mucocutaneous 43
  mucous membranes 43, 48
  nodule 44, 49–52
  oesophagus 43
  oropharynx 43
  pleural 50
  pulmonary 51
  rectal 49
  stomach 43, 49
  treatment 58
  visceral involvement 43, 49
Ketoconazole 95

Lanceolate diplococci 69
LAV 10, 20
Leucopenia 99
Leukaemia 10
Leukoencephalopathy
  progressive multifocal
    (PML) 2, 74, 80–87
Leukopenia 38
Lethargy 78
Lichen planus 44
Lymphadenopathy 24, 26
  associated virus see LAV
  persistent generalized see
    PGL
Lymphocyte
  CD4+ 7, 8, 42
    central role of 9
    cultures 17
  CD8+ 42
Lymphoid
  interstitial
    pneumonia 2, 3, 23
    pneumonitis 60
  neoplasia
    extracranial 55
Lymphoma 27, 55–57, 85
  cerebral 23, 55, 56
  CNS 74, 78

Hodgkin's 56
malignant 57
non-Hodgkin's 55, 56
systemic 74
Lymphomas 1, 78
Lymph node
biopsy 26, 27
involvement 27
Lymphopenia 7, 38, 42

Macule 44
Macrophage 8–9, 19
Malabsorption 85
Megakaryocytes 40
Memory loss 75
Meningeal irritation 76
Meningitis 74
aseptic 24–25, 76
cryptococcal 74–75, 78,
82–83
Meningoencephalitis 83
Metallic taste 92
Metronidazole 37
Miconazole 95
Microabscesses
multiple 83
Microglial cells 19

β_2-microglobulin
increase of 42
Microsporidia 85
Molluscum contagiosum 28,
34, 35
Monocyte function 7
Monocytes 19
Mononeuropathies
multiple 74
Myalgia 101
Mycobacteria 71
atypical 60, 71
Mycobacterial
infection 67
infections 27, 38
Mycobacterium tuberculosis
disseminated 39
extrapulmonary 3

Mycobacterium avium
disseminated 2
intracellulare 67
Mycobacterium kansasii
disseminated 2
Mycobacterium xenopi 61, 71
Myopathy 23–25, 75
vacuolar 76

Naevi 44
Nausea 92–93, 95, 101
Necrosis
frontal and temporal
lobes   81
Neoplasia 85
extracranial lymphoid 55
Neurological
complications 74
disease 23
signs 78, 83
syndromes 24, 76
Neuropathies
cranial 74
Neuropathy
inflammatory
demyelinating 74
peripheral 23
sensory 74
Neuropsychological testing 75
Neurosyphilis 74–75
Neutropenia 38, 42, 94
Nerve palsies
cranial 76
Night sweats 27, 60
Nystatin 95
Oedema
cerebral 78
facial 48
lobes
frontal, temporal 81
penis 49
scrotum 49

Opportunistic infections
1, 43, 60–95
disseminated 38
major 23

minor 27, 30
treatment
    fungal 95
    protozoal 92–93
    viral 94
'Owl's eye'
    cell 65–66
    inclusion 89

P24 antigen assay 16
Paediatric
    patient groups USA 4
    cases, in USA 5
Pain
    abdominal 88–89
    chest 62
Pancytopenia 38, 103
Papovavirus 80
Papilloma virus, human
    28, 34–35, 58
Paraesthesia 76
Patient groups, USA 4
Pentamidine 92, 93
Periodontis 28, 37
PGL 23, 26–27, 29, 34, 38,
    40, 68
Phosphonoformate 98
Pityriasis versicolor 28
Pneumococcal pneumonia 69
Pneumococcus 60
Pneumocystis carinii
    cysts 63, 64
    maintenance 93
    pneumonia 1–3, 59, 60, 62–65
    treatment 92
    trophozoites 63
Pneumonitis
    interstitial 73
Polyneuropathy 76
Pox virus 34
Progression
    risk of 41–42
Proliferative responses 7
Pseudomonas aeruginosa 68
Psoriasis 28, 30, 35
Pulmonary syndrome 60–61
Purpura 40

Purpuric rash 41
Pyremethamine 93
Pyrexias 60

Quinine 93

Radiotherapy 53
Rash 24, 92–93
    diffuse macular 24
    purpuric 41
Release signs 75
Replication
    HIV 97
    viral 19
Retrosternal discomfort/
    dysphagia 85
Ribavirin 98
Rifamycin derivatives 98

Salmonella 85
    septicaemia 3
Seborrhoeic dermatitis 28–29
Seizures 78, 81–82
Seroconversion illness 24
Seroepidemiology 1
Shadowing
    bilateral alveolar/
        interstitial 62
    normal 62
    patchy 71
SIV 20
Skin 28
    anergy 7
    dry 28
    lesions
        Kaposi's sarcoma
        43, 45–49
Spiramycin 93
Splenectomy 40
Sputum
    mucoid 62
    purulent 62
    mycobacterial 67
Steroids
    in treatment 40
STLV-III 20
Streptococcus Pneumoniae 68

Syphilis
  secondary 44

Thrombocytopenia 24, 95
  autoimmune 40–41
Tinea cruris 32–33
  pedis/coporis/other 28
Toxoplasma cyst 80
Toxoplasmosis
  cerebral 2, 3, 56, 74,
    78–80
    features of 78
Treatment
  candidiasis 95
  cryptococcosis 95
  cryptosporidium 85, 88–89
  cytomegalovirus (CMV) 94
  Herpes simplex 94
  Herpes zoster 23, 33
  Isosporiasis 93
  Kaposi's carcoma 53
  opportunistic infections
    92–95
  Pneumocystis carinii 92
  toxoplasmosis 93
Trimethoprim 92
Tumour necrosis factor 99
Tumors 1, 23, 43, 58–59
  anogenital tract 58
  oral cavity 58

Ulceration
  perianal 85, 90–91

Vaccines 104–107
Varicella zoster 28, 30, 91
Villous atrophy 87
Vomiting 95, 101
Violaceous plaque 44

Warts 34
Warts
  anorectal 85
Wasting 87
Weakness 76
Weight loss 27, 55, 60–61, 85
Western blot 21

Zidovudine 39–40, 96,
  98, 100–103

NOTES

NOTES

NOTES

NOTES

NOTES

NOTES